ARTHRITIS

How allergy may aggravate or even cause arthritis

By the same author

THE MIGRAINE REVOLUTION

Also for arthritis sufferers:

NEW SELF HELP ARTHRITIS
A DOCTOR'S NEW HOME CURE FOR ARTHRITIS
DIETS TO HELP ARTHRITIS

ARTHRITIS

The Allergy Connection

Dr John Mansfield

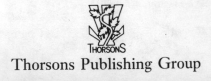

Thorsons Publishing Group

First published 1990

Copyright © John Mansfield 1990

British Library Cataloguing in Publication Data

Mansfield, John
Arthritis: the allergy connection.
1. Man. Joints. Arthritis
I. Title
616.7′22

ISBN 0 7225 1903 6

*Published by Thorsons Publishers Limited, Wellingborough,
Northamptonshire NN8 2RQ, England*

Printed in Great Britain by Mackays of Chatham, Kent

1 3 5 7 9 10 8 6 4 2

Contents

Foreword   7

Introduction   9

1 Three case histories of arthritis   15

2 Food allergy and arthritis   21

3 Chemical sensitivity and arthritis   43

4 Alcohol and smoking in relation to arthritis   52

5 Inhaled allergies and arthritis   58

6 Intestinal candidiasis   64

7 Psoriatic arthritis and ankylosing spondylitis   85

8 Different clinical types of arthritis   93

9 The elimination diet   102

10 Neutralization and desensitization to foods   131

11 Neutralization to inhalants and chemicals   144

12 Clinical trials of allergy and rheumatoid arthritis   149

13 Clinical trials of neutralization   159

14 The roots of allergy   168

15 The language and philosophy of New Medicine 177

Summary 185

Index 190

Foreword

I remember well my introduction to food allergy. Two patients with painful joints I had been looking after had failed to improve despite everything I could think of and both fortunately had the good sense to look elsewhere. After attending Dr Mansfield's clinic, they both very kindly contacted me to say that if they avoided particular foods, they remained well.

Thus started my own interest in the ideas and approaches you will read about in this book. While some will not benefit, there is certainly no doubt that many more will, from following the sorts of approach described. While some of the things discussed could be considered controversial, the more appropriate description of much in this book is 'exciting' or 'interesting', or even 'quite fascinating'. As someone who has spent many years learning about and prescribing drugs with quite variable benefit and lots of potential side-effects, it has been most gratifying to see patients with painful, swollen joints lose their pain and swelling, simply by avoiding particular foods. What is most interesting of all is the possibility that something in these foods is not just aggravating a condition such as rheumatoid arthritis, but perhaps even causing it, and in the long-term treatment of this condition finding and removing the cause remains the ultimate goal.

As Dr Mansfield emphasizes, however, this approach is not limited to a consideration of the role that food reactions may play in these conditions. Chemicals, inhaled allergens, and the flora of the intestines can all play a part in some people.

This book deserves to be widely read, not just by people with painful joints but also by the doctors who look after them. It should be read by researchers so that much more effort is directed towards finding out just what it is in foods that makes joints sore, and directed towards drug companies so that effort is aimed more towards removing underlying causes of arthritis rather than suppressing symptoms.

Dr Jeff Reardon MB, MRCP
Consultant in Rheumatology & Rehabilitation
Mayday Hospital, Croydon, Surrey

Introduction

You may be surprised that arthritis has any connection with allergy at all. Surely allergy means hay fever, runny noses, asthma, and certain skin disorders? There is, however, an enormous body of evidence which shows that almost all forms of arthritis, including rheumatoid arthritis, non-specific arthritis, osteoarthritis, and psoriatic arthritis, are related to allergy, intolerance, or hypersensitivity to various environmental factors. These factors can be food, chemicals in food, the chemicals we breathe, or the allergenic particles which we inhale, such as house dust, house dust mites, or moulds.

The exciting consequence of this is that, if this is so for you, by identifying these factors, you can become free of arthritis. Sometimes this can be accompanied by the simple avoidance of specific foods, but sometimes avoidance of air-borne allergens or multiple food allergens is impossible and specific neutralization therapy may be needed instead. I do not include in this category those rare forms of arthritis such as viral arthritis, septic arthritis, or rheumatic fever which are, as is well understood, caused by specific viruses or bacteria.

This concept is not just theory: there are nowadays many thousands of people in the United Kingdom, the United States of America, Canada, and Australia walking around free or almost free of the arthritic pain and swelling that used to ruin their lives.

Some of these people (the luckier ones) have found relief after reading one of a number of popular books on the market giving specific dietary advice to arthritic sufferers. Typical of these, and in my opinion one of the better ones, is Dr G. W. Campbell's book *A Doctor's Proven New Home Cure for Arthritis*, published in the UK by Thorsons. This book advocates eating exclusively, for one week, foods that you rarely consume and this will often lead to a major improvement in the arthritic symptoms. By slowly reintroducing everyday foods into the diet you can observe which foods re-create the arthritic problem. Dr Campbell also recognizes the problem of chemicals in foods and adds appropriate advice about this problem.

Some arthritic sufferers who have simple allergy problems confined to the area of food are helped by this method, though many are not because they are more complicated. Those that respond, and I have met a number of them, often gleefully report the spectacular improvement to their GP or rheumatologist. On many occasions their observations are met with total disbelief and the physicians invoke the explanation of 'spontaneous remission' to explain the improvement. These physicians, amazingly, seem uninterested by the patient's offer to re-eat the 'bad' foods and demonstrate an abrupt end to this spontaneous remission for a few days. Some physicians have very little curiosity about such potentially earth-shaking phenomena. Most patients give up trying to interest their physicians and thereby to help millions of sufferers who need similar help.

The reason that many people are not helped by simple dietary manipulation is that many have more complicated food sensitivities, possibly further complicated by reactions to inhaled allergens or ingested chemicals. In some people, reactions to inhaled allergens such as house dust, house dust mites, and moulds are very important (consider how often arthritis is made significantly worse just before a thunderstorm when the mould count in the atmosphere increases enormously).

In extremely complicated cases one can demonstrate that the arthritic problem is allergic by placing sufferers in a totally allergy-free environment where they fast for a few days. There are two such clinics, called environmental control clinics, in the UK, and several in the USA. It is uncommon for patients to enter such a clinic and not lose most of their arthritic symptoms in six days while fasting and despite no medication unless they have irreversibly damaged joints. Staff in these clinics routinely observe arthritic patients losing their symptoms in a few days and any physician working in such a clinic can hardly fail to conclude that arthritis is a condition caused by environmental factors.

Observations in these clinics show that common forms of arthritis are *not* caused by a mythical virus. They are, furthermore, *not* caused by auto-immunity, i.e. the body becoming allergic to itself. Auto-immunity has been postulated in the past as many of the changes in the blood of sufferers from rheumatoid arthritis suggest an allergic or immune process is going on. As food sensitivity has never been seriously considered by many, the idea that one is reacting to one's own body has gained ground.

Well over 90 per cent of people who do not have irreversibly damaged joints improve spectacularly in the environmental units, but a few don't. Some of these have had their immune systems so battered and compromised by years of taking potent cortisone-derived drugs that the condition appears to have become irreversible, despite the removal of the main precipitating factors. It would seem that the immune system of these individuals has become incapable of re-asserting itself under any circumstances. A few sufferers appear to react to organisms in their bowel, particularly one called Candida albicans, commonly known as thrush. Such people are not helped by entering an environmental unit and fasting. They can, however, be treated by other means and Chapter 6 relates to this problem.

The vast majority of people, however, do not need the attention of an environmental control unit and its attendant expense. They can normally be helped by attending an outpatient clinic specializing in this approach. In-depth history taking will often yield clues as to whether the problems relate to food, chemicals, or other, inhaled allergens. Elimination diets and skin-testing using the intradermal provocative technique (see Chapters 9, 10 and 11) further elucidate the problem. Although there are several hundred such clinics in the USA, there are only about twelve in the UK. They are known to organizations such as Action Against Allergy, set up to promote interest and research into the allergic basis of illness. These organizations, of which there are several, are listed at the end of this book.

Many readers, especially physicians, are bound to be pretty sceptical about what I am saying and this is only right and proper. There has, however, been a great deal of research to substantiate these claims and several carefully controlled clinical trials have been reported in reputable journals. To British doctors, perhaps the most interesting one was that done by my own clinic in conjunction with the Department of Rheumatology at Epsom District Hospital. This was a single-blind placebo-controlled trial of dietary manipulative therapy in classical rheumatoid arthritis. The trial was designed by one of the leading trial designers in the UK and was published in *The*

Lancet in February 1986. Papers are not accepted by *The Lancet* unless the trial has been conducted in the highest possible scientific manner. This trial is detailed with others in Chapter 12. Briefly, although at the time we restricted our attention to food sensitivity, 75 per cent of the 44 patients involved in the trial responded well or totally. An American trial taking into account all factors and performed within three environmental control units came up with better results still, as was to be expected.

The purpose of this book is to inform physicians and arthritis sufferers of the possibilities of this approach. Many readers will be desperately seeking a solution to their problems, and although private out-patient care is not normally very expensive (usually in toto about the cost of a clutch replacement in a large family car), many cannot afford this. Accordingly I have included a self-help step-by-step elimination diet in Chapter 9 so that those people may be able to sort out their own problems.

In practice, though, most people do better if they have a physician to guide them through the various pitfalls that can occur on the way, particularly if they have a large number of allergies. Ultimately, even those who do manage to identify the cause of their problems may nevertheless have to seek a physician's help as the foods implicated are often such basic ingredients of the Western diet as wheat, corn, milk, eggs, yeast, cane sugar, beet sugar, and soy. All these items are of course very difficult to avoid and are often hidden ingredients in complex foods. Desensitization to these foods by the intradermal provocative neutralization technique described in Chapters 9, 10 and 11 may be necessary to enable such individuals to eat reasonably normally.

Summing up, therefore, I am stating that:

- Most forms of arthritis are environmentally induced.
- There are techniques available for sorting out which environmental components are important in each individual.
- There is clinical evidence of the validity of this approach in the shape of:

    a) many thousands of people who have been relieved of their problems
    b) scientifically controlled clinical trials published in learned medical journals.

- This approach to arthritis represents just one aspect of a new approach to illness which has demonstrated that much chronic illness is related to individual reactions between the human organism and its environment. The approach has been variously called 'Allergy and Environmental Medicine', 'Nutri-allergy', 'Clinical Ecology', and, because none of these terms is entirely satisfactory to cover the whole field, maybe more simply 'New Medicine'.

Drug therapy

The need for an approach like this is particularly vital in view of the unsatisfactory situation in regard to drug therapy with arthritis. The first-line approach to the arthritic problem, irrespective of the form of arthritis, is either aspirin or the non-steroidal anti-inflammatory drugs. Aspirin has well-known gastric side-effects taken in large dosage and all the non-steroidal anti-inflammatory drugs have a very high incidence of side-effects. Some, of which Opren is the most notorious, have been demonstrated to have horrific side-effects and have been totally withdrawn from the market. None of these drugs eradicates arthritis or even beneficially changes its progress. There has even been a report in *The Sunday Times* containing evidence collected by Dr Paul Dieppe of Bristol University that this category of drugs could lead to a prolongation of the disease process. In other words, it appears that these drugs could inhibit the natural healing processes that tend to occur in the normal situation.

The other drugs used, particularly for rheumatoid arthritis, are the disease-modifying drugs, such as Cortisone, Penicillamine, and Gold. These can beneficially alter the course of the disease but they are all very potent drugs with a high incidence of side-effects and occasional fatalities. These drugs are normally employed only with the more desperate patients because of the risks involved, and one rheumatologist I know was stimulated into adopting the allergic approach to arthritis as a result of the death of one of his patients after Gold injections.

Hippocrates, the father of medicine, instructed physicians that above all else they should not do harm to their patients. The non-drug approach I am advocating has never caused serious harm to anyone.

1 Three case histories of arthritis

It seems appropriate at this point to relate three separate examples of cases I have treated which illustrate some of the problems that we meet when we attempt to diagnose the factors that contribute to arthritis. Having applied these techniques to over 2,000 cases of arthritis, I found it difficult to select three but finally decided on one case of osteoarthritis that was quite easy to sort out, one case of non-specific arthritis that was moderately difficult, and one extremely severe case of rheumatoid arthritis that was incredibly complex. The first two cases are typical of everyday experience but the third one is quite unusual and extraordinary.

Tony G.

The first case we will call Tony G. The magazine *Here's Health* had reported several cases of arthritis sufferers who had done very well using allergy detection techniques, and they rang me to ask if they could send a patient to the clinic and follow his progress through the elimination diet or other tests that we would use. I thought this was an interesting challenge.

When Tony, a dairy farmer, first consulted me he was 58 years old. He had in the preceding two or three years suffered increasing pain, swelling and stiffening, especially in the hands, wrists, and knees. There was a small degree of the same problem in his hips and shoulders. He had seen his GP on several occasions, and a rheumatologist. As a result of blood tests and examinations by these doctors, he had been diagnosed as suffering from osteoarthritis.

After taking his history and finding no specific indication of chemical or inhalant sensitivity, I elected to put him on a low-risk (allergy-wise) diet for 6½ days. In this time he limited his diet to four round fish (cod, trout, salmon and mackerel), carrots, pears, courgettes, marrow, parsnips, turnips, swedes, and sweet potatoes. The only fluid we allowed was bottled spring water and the only condiment was sea salt.

On the first three days of this diet, Tony had the classic and normal withdrawal response and felt rather worse than usual, but by the seventh day when he reattended my clinic he was able to report a spectacular improvement (about 90 per cent) in all his joints. The only residual symptom at this point was some stiffness in his hands and a little pain in one index finger. It must be emphasized that he was on no drugs of any kind while on the diet and the improvement on the diet decidedly exceeded any he had ever noticed with drugs.

Tony then embarked on a programme of reintroducing foods into the diet. At this point I was sure, because of the great improvement, that his arthritis was related to food sensitivity, but we now had to find out which foods were implicated in his particular case. When a food has not been eaten for over five days it will produce a perceivable reaction when reintroduced into the diet, as long as there has been a major improvement in the symptoms. In the next five weeks Tony had the following 'reactions':

tap water:	four hours later, pain in his fingers and right hand, swollen knuckles; other joints remained satisfactory.
wheat:	pain and swelling in all his joints within 12 hours: these symptoms took three days to disperse.
malt:	pain and swelling again in his hands and fingers within 24 hours, and this reaction took two days to disappear.

These three items were then retested after a minimum of five days' avoidance and all three clearly reacted again on the second test.

The tap water reaction was probably the most interesting: we discovered that Tony was reacting to the chlorine component in the tap water. We discovered this by observing that he did not react to tap water which had been boiled for several minutes. Chlorine is volatile and is about the only substance removed by boiling. Tony had been using concentrated chlorine for many years for sterilizing his dairy equipment and this practice had probably sensitized him to the chlorine. Once sensitized, he then reacted to the small amounts of chlorine found in ordinary tap water.

Reaction to grains such as wheat and malt is very common in arthritic sufferers and as they are difficult to avoid we employed 'neutralization therapy' to enable Tony to eat these foods without adverse effect. This technique is described in Chapters 10 and 11 and, using it, Tony has remained free of his arthritis in the subsequent few years, but has managed to continue eating wheat and malt. He has been able to continue his farming, which of course is a fairly physical job, and run up and down stairs with no problem, in marked contrast to the situation prior to his allergy work-out.

He could, if he wished, avoid wheat and malt, but the neutralization treatment involves only one small neutralizing injection taken every two or three days that immediately enables him to eat the food to which he is sensitive. After about three years the injections become unnecessary and the individual is then completely cured of his specific food sensitivity.

Irene A.

The second case I have selected is Irene A., a middle-aged woman of Swiss descent. She lived with her husband in a lovely country village in Surrey. She was the patient of a local GP, Dr B., who had an interest in the allergy and environmental approach to illness. As he was also a Postgraduate Organizer he had heard several of my lectures to young doctors about to enter general practice.

Irene had multiple severe joint pains and swelling, and she had consulted some of the most eminent rheumatologists, both in Switzerland and in London. As there were none of the characteristic blood changes of rheumatoid arthritis, she had been diagnosed as suffering from non-specific arthritis and she was a particularly severe case of this. The arthritis was so severe that she had been taking Cortisone tablets for 1½ years and in addition had had multiple Cortisone injections into the various affected joints. When she returned from Switzerland once to see her general practitioner she was in the quite desperate state of having had five years of painful misery with absolutely no end in sight.

Dr B. decided to put Irene on a diet of about five foods with a low risk of allergy. On this diet she had a severe withdrawal reaction with increased symptoms in the first three or four days, but by the sixth day there was the most spectacular improvement in her joint pains. On reintroducing foods into the diet Irene had severe responses to orange, lemon, grapefruit, wine vinegar, and raspberries. The reaction to orange was extremely severe and lasted for three days. Interestingly, Irene used to drink orange juice at least every morning and used lemon prolifically in all her cooking.

After Dr B. had completed the elimination diet Irene felt at least 70 per cent improved. However, after completing the elimination diet she went to visit her mother in Zurich, Switzerland. Within a couple of days of staying at the flat in Zurich she was delighted to find that her joints had improved to 100 per cent. Assuming this to be a late benefit of Dr B.'s dietary investigation, she could hardly wait to return to England to tell him of her improvement. To her dismay, when she later returned to her Surrey home, many of the joint pains returned within 48 hours. She reported her experiences to Dr B., who concluded that there must be an environmental factor other than food sensitivity in her problems and sent her to my clinic.

On our first consultation it was fairly obvious to me that she was reacting to household gas. The flat in Zurich was all-electric, but her Surrey home had a gas cooker and gas-fired central heating with the boiler situated in the kitchen. Skin-testing showed that she was sensitive to gas and so we advised a trial in which all her gas utilities were turned off at the mains. She was also advised to make sure that the house was well-ventilated. Within a few days of this being done, Irene's joints were as good as they had been in Switzerland. On re-establishing her gas utilities she suffered a return of the arthritis within 24-48 hours. She was by now more than convinced about the role that the gas was playing in her problems and she sold her gas cooker and replaced it with an electric one. The gas central heating boiler was moved to an outhouse so that the gas was burnt outside the confines of the house. This of course cost several hundred pounds but was probably the best money that Irene has ever spent. These events all occurred over five years ago and she has had no recurrence of symptoms since that time.

To an independent observer, the most compelling feature of this case, and why I have included it, is the sheer accidental way that the patient stumbled over the final answer to her problems. We are always testing patients for environmental factors and making appropriate changes if necessary. Rarely do these discoveries occur by accident as they did in her case.

Joe E.

When Joe E. initially attended my clinic he was 24 years old. He was extremely severely affected with what had been diagnosed as partly rheumatoid arthritis and partly ankylosing spondylitis. The problems with his joints had started when he was 14. By the following year, the joint pains were quite severe, and complicated by psychological problems such as depression which became very severe at times; he bordered on suicide on these days. There were in addition problems with allergic reactions to the drugs which he was prescribed for his arthritis. Joc also had rhinitis (runny nose), and prick skin-tests had shown him to be sensitive to allergens such as house dust and house dust mite.

I will never forget the day that Joe first arrived at the clinic. He was unable to walk so his father lifted him into my consulting room and laid him on the couch. He looked extremely ill and emaciated. His feet were so swollen that he was wearing carpet slippers several sizes larger than his real foot size. What Joe had discovered for himself, after reading books on the subject and before he attended my clinic, was that if he fasted for a few days there was an enormous reduction in his joint pain and swelling. However, to his distress, he could only find about two foods which would not immediately cause his symptoms to recur in severe form within a matter of hours.

With such a history I felt that, although food sensitivity was clearly important in Joe's case, there was little point in trying an elimination diet. Accordingly we embarked on an ambitious programme of neutralization therapy. First we selected about 30 foods which Joe would be happy to eat and skin-tested him to each one. As expected he reacted to all of them. He had positive skin wheal reactions on the stronger strengths accompanied by symptoms, followed by relief of symptoms when we discovered the weaker neutralizing dose. Taking a cocktail of all his neutralizing doses in one single injection on alternate days, and restricting his diet to the foods covered by the injection, produced an enormous improvement in his joint pains within a few days.

Knowing Joe was sensitive to inhaled allergens such as house dust and house dust mite but not knowing what symptoms these allergies were producing, we skin-tested for these and found the appropriate neutralizing levels. To our delight, when he took these injections in addition to his food injections there was a further quantum improvement in the condition of his joints.

A few days after Joe had taken a combination of the food and inhalant injections his mother, who had stood by Joe in all his tribulations, rang excitedly to tell me that he had just come back from a three-mile walk, the first that he had accomplished for many years. Further skin-testing revealed some chemical sensitivities, and some modification to the house and the chemicals found there produced even more improvement. Joe, therefore, appeared to have developed a sensitivity to almost everything in his environment. Such pan-sensitivities are quite rare but these results showed that, even in this extraordinary type of case, help can be given using neutralization therapy.

Within a few months of starting treatment Joe was back at work and living independently in his fourth-floor flat in London (64 steps up). He continued to take neutralizing injections for a few years and occasionally went a bit 'off-colour', a situation which was quickly remedied by adjusting his neutralizing levels. He has remained very well right up to the present day and has developed a successful career in the world of graphic art. Anyone meeting him in the past few years would never guess at the agonies that beset him between the ages of 14 and 24, as now he is entirely well in every respect.

2 Food allergy and arthritis

The idea that foods can produce abnormal reactions has a long history and has always been the subject of considerable medical interest. The aphorism 'one man's meat is another man's poison' has been attributed to Lucretius, who lived about 100 years BC. For many centuries, dietary manipulations were one of the main areas of medical endeavour, but as interest in pharmacology grew in the last century this concept was relegated to the backwaters of medicine. It has recently been demonstrated that this was a considerable oversight.

Individual case reports of differing types of arthritis being related to food allergy have appeared in medical literature extending as far back as 1917. However, the first physician to draw attention in a big way to the inter-relationship of food allergy and arthritis was Dr Michael Zeller, who was a clinical instructor in medicine at the University of Illinois College of Medicine in Chicago. He wrote a paper published in 1948 in the *Annals of Allergy* entitled 'Rheumatoid Arthritis: Food Allergy as a Factor'. In this paper Dr Zeller strongly emphasized his observations that symptoms of arthritis could frequently be relieved by appropriate food exclusion diets. The subsequent reproduction of arthritic symptoms on reingestion of certain foods established the cause of that patient's rheumatoid arthritis. Repeated reintroductions of identified food allergens with a minimum of five-day intervals could be shown to reproduce the arthritis response on each occasion. Zeller realized that not all cases of rheumatoid arthritis were due entirely to food allergy and all subsequent serious investigators have found the same.

Another major contributor to this concept at about the same time was Dr Albert Rowe. Dr Rowe lived in California and was an emeritus Lecturer in Medicine at the University of California in San Francisco. He discovered early in his career that food allergy was a major cause of many illnesses and that trying to diagnose it by ordinary skin prick tests was quite useless. He devised complex exclusion dietary procedures which led to the complete relief of symptoms in countless people. He established a very high reputation and patients flooded to see him from all over the world.

Dr Rowe was a prolific writer and first published his book *Food Allergy* in 1931. There is a whole chapter on food allergy and arthritis, which cites many case histories illustrating relief of various forms of arthritis as a result of exclusion diets. Dr Rowe also emphasized the necessity of reintroducing foods into the diet to identify the foods which were responsible for the arthritis pain in each individual.

Dr Theron Randolph of Chicago, Illinois, who in his early career was an instructor in medicine at North Western University Medical School in Chicago, was a close acquaintance of Dr Michael Zeller and was well acquainted with Dr Albert Rowe's work in California. Dr Randolph's enormous contribution to medicine was the discovery that, when rigid dietary exclusion was carried out in a chemically free and allergy-free environment, *almost all cases responded dramatically.*

From this discovery was born the idea of comprehensive environmental control in purpose-built clinics. These environmental control units are built of hard materials that do not give off chemical odours (in the USA this is known as 'out-gassing'). Solid materials such as glass, concrete, metals, porcelainized steel, mosaic tiles, marble, etc. are utilized in their construction. The interiors are equipped with materials such as pure cotton which have no chemical contaminant. The air is filtered prior to entering the unit, to remove dusts, atmospheric moulds, and chemical pollutants, and it is blown into the unit under pressure. No gas or fossil fuels are burnt inside the unit, and perfumes, deodorants, cigarettes, etc. are strictly banned. Food used in these units are organically derived, as people can react to the contaminants of foods (pesticides, insecticides, colourants, preservatives, etc.) as well as to the foods themselves. All these factors will be discussed in much more detail in later chapters.

Defining allergy

Returning now to the food allergy component, it is probably at this point appropriate to clarify the term 'allergy' itself. In 1906 an Austrian physician called Clement von Pirquet coined the term from two Greek words which meant 'altered reactivity'. In other words, an allergy was a response to a substance which affected one individual but not another. Allergy therefore contrasts with toxicity. Toxicity affects everyone, though usually to varying degrees. Everyone is killed with hydrogen cyanide but only some people react adversely to milk. About 1906 it was beginning to be realized that many illnesses were an inter-reaction between environmental factors and susceptible individuals, and the term 'allergy' described this situation well.

The use or misuse of the term has caused the most amazing schisms among physicians working with patients who have adverse reactions to foods. Most immunologists assert that when von Pirquet coined the term 'allergy' he meant it to cover only those reactions in which a specific immunologic (antigen-antibody) reaction could be determined. A colleague of von Pirquet, Dr Doerr, in a paper published in 1909, quite definitely widened the use of the term to cover every form of altered reactivity, whether an underlying antigen-antibody reaction could be shown or not.

Close study of von Pirquet's writings showed he realized that immune reactions and supersensitivities can be most closely related and often impossible to dissociate. He thus meant 'allergy' to be a term which would prejudice nothing and could cover reactions which had no known immunologic basis. Because of this I use the word freely throughout this text.

The year 1925 was an historic one in the field of allergy, but for those physicians taking a wide view of allergy an 'infamous' one. Interest in food allergy had just started to grow, particularly in the USA. However, in 1925, European and British allergists persuaded their American colleagues to restrict their definition of allergy to those mechanisms which could be explained by the antigen-antibody hypothesis. This of course made the field extremely 'scientific'. These reactions could be measured accurately in the laboratory and did not depend on the involvement of such unpredictable factors as actual patients and their own observations! The most eminent American immunologist of the day, Arthur F. Coca of Cornell University, fought strongly against this restrictive view, but most of his colleagues in the allergy profession went along with this new orthodoxy. The last 20 years, however, has seen the emergence of many physicians in North America, Great Britain, and Australia who have reported countless cases of non-immunologic allergy and their work has re-challenged this narrow view of allergy. Many immunologically orientated physicians have now come round to the same viewpoint, although there is still resistance from some of the immunologic establishment.

Masked food allergy

Perhaps the most important single fact to grasp about food allergy is the concept of 'masking'. Most people are familiar with and understand the idea that someone can consume an occasionally eaten food and feel ill afterwards. Because of this, the public concept of food allergy has mostly been related to occasionally eaten and exotic foods. Many physicians also take this simplistic view of food allergy.

Dr Rowe in his early days did not understand masking and he noted there was a difference between immediate and delayed reactions, but he had not discovered that what would normally be a delayed reaction could be converted into an immediate one if the food were omitted from the diet for at least five days. When a food is reintroduced in these circumstances the reaction usually occurs within four or five hours, except for slowly absorbed foods such as cereals.

The concept of masked food allergy was originally identified by Dr Herbert Rinkel, a well-known allergist practising in Oklahoma City. Dr Rinkel was renowned for being an extremely acute observer of various cause and effect relationships. After he qualified in medicine, he developed a severe nasal allergy called an allergic rhinitis, which is a condition characterized by severe persistent nasal discharge. His medical colleagues skin-tested him for all the well-known inhalant allergies and these test proved negative.

Dr Rinkel was familiar with Dr Rowe's work on food allergy and suspected he might have such a problem himself. When he had been a medical student, like many of his colleagues, he had been fairly impecunious. Grants are not common in the USA and, generally speaking, medical students going through college there have to support themselves or be supported by their parents. Rinkel's father, who was an egg farmer, had supported his son during his medical studentship by sending him a gross of eggs (144) each week and this was the main source of protein for Rinkel and his family. This high ingestion of eggs continued after he qualified and he therefore suspected eggs as a cause of his problem. One afternoon, in an attempt to produce an adverse reaction, he consumed a large quantity of eggs, but to his surprise his nasal symptoms in that afternoon were, if anything, rather improved. Some years later he did the opposite – he abstained from eggs for about five days and then discovered that his nasal discharge improved very considerably. After five days he inadvertently consumed some angel cake (which of course contains egg) at a birthday party. He suddenly collapsed unconscious and his rhinitis returned in dramatic fashion.

Dr Rinkel conceived as a result of this experience that he might well have stumbled on something fundamental regarding the basic nature of food allergy. He thus repeated the experiment by re-establishing his consumption of eggs, omitting them again for five days and again repeating the egg ingestion, which caused a recurrence of the symptoms of unconsciousness and nasal discharge. He next extended his observations to a number of his patients and found a similar phenomenon occurring with a wide variety of different foods and with a wide variety of medical conditions, including joint pain. His observations were first published in 1944, where masking was defined in the following way: if a person ingests a particular food each day he or she may become allergic to it and yet not suspect this as a cause of the symptoms. It is usual to feel better after a meal than before. In this case the feedings tend to mask the symptoms of the allergic response. Dr Rinkel could not explain his observations.

Since Dr Rinkel's original work, cases of masked food allergy have been reported in many thousands of patients. Masked food allergy represents an interesting model of addictive behaviour and is, in my opinion, the major basic mechanism behind the addition to such apparently diverse items as coffee, tea, sugar, alcoholic beverages, and tobacco. This concept can be represented graphically, as shown in Figure 1.

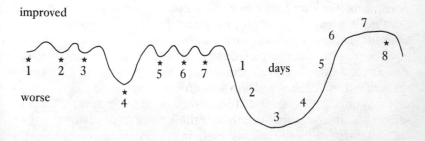

Figure 1   Masked food allergy

This graph illustrates the results of eating or not eating a masked food allergen in someone with a single food allergy. Each asterisk represents the feeding of the allergenic food. As can be seen, the second feeding aborts the deterioration of symptoms which is seen after the first feeding. This is followed by an improvement. A similar response is experienced after the third feeding. Because the fourth feeding of the allergenic food is delayed, the response is further down the withdrawal curve and is thus worse. Following this fourth feeding, the person's condition usually returns to normal.

After the seventh feeding, in this example, the subject has been told to avoid the allergenic food and then exhibits the classic withdrawal phenomenon, characterized by a considerable deterioration of symptoms, usually by the evening of the first day. These symptoms may be of joint pain, headache, or fatigue. The second and third day tend to be quite severe, but they are followed by a slow improvement until the sixth day. By the sixth day most people are symptom-free if under 35 years old. In those who are older than 35, the symptoms may take another day or so to clear. It is extremely gratifying to see someone with constant arthritis pain clear of symptoms for the first time for several years on the sixth or seventh day of this withdrawal period. Feeding after the seventh day (* 8) represents a deliberate re-feeding of the avoided food and the Rinkel hyperacute response. In this, as illustrated by Rinkel's experience, symptoms return quickly and quite dramatically.

Figure 1 demonstrates how complicated is the relationship between one commonly-eaten food allergen and the symptomatology that it creates. Imagine, therefore, if one is dealing with a patient who has allergies to wheat, corn, milk, and yeast, there will be a different curve of symptomatology for each food depending on the frequency at which it is eaten. Any relationship between food and symptoms will in these circumstances become far from obvious. I emphasize this point because many physicians believe that if food allergy is present, it will be obvious to all those concerned. It is partly this simplistic view of the subject which has led to its neglect.

The concept of masking is the single most important factor to grasp about the inter-relationship of food and arthritis. It explains why so many arthritis patients feel so bad first thing in the morning. Many of them think it is the immobility of the night's sleep and the subsequent stiffness that this might engender. There may be an element of this but mostly it is the non-consumption of the foods to which they are sensitive. Arthritis patients often also feel worse if they happen to miss their breakfast which normally contains one of the foods to which they are sensitive.

The concept of masking also explains why some foods eaten only on an occasional and intermittent basis are known by certain people to worsen their arthritis. When I talk to arthritis patients a surprising number know that a certain occasionally eaten food may produce some worsening of their symptoms, although obviously other factors are operating, as avoidance of this food does not eliminate the problem. Patients often mention these observations to rheumatologists who by and large ignore them.

Unfortunately these observations, which were originally made 40 years ago, were ignored or misunderstood by the medical profession in general, but a full account of the concept was given in what is now the classic textbook on the subject: *Food Allergy* by Herbert J. Rinkel MD, Theron G. Randolph MD, and Michael Zeller MD. It was originally published in 1951 by Charles C. Thomas in the USA, but because of the current explosion of interest in this field, it has been republished by The New England Foundation for Allergic and Environmental Diseases of the Alan Mandell Centre for Bio-Ecologic Diseases. In that book the main basic concepts of food allergy are described in great detail.

Adaptation

An allergy represents the failure of an organism to adapt to its environment. Much human illness, therefore, stems from the inability of the human organism to adapt to new foods or chemicals brought into the environment, or an overdosage of such items. The original concept of adaptation was first described by Hans Selye, an eminent physiologist working at McGill University in Montreal. In 1936 Selye's work was published in the journal, *Nature*, entitled 'The General Adaptation Syndrome'. He described the Adaptation Syndrome as a characteristic set of events which could be produced by a wide range of harmful agents. He stated that experiments on rats showed that if the organism is severely damaged by acute non-specific harmful agents (such as exposure to cold, surgical injury, excessive muscular exercise, or intoxication with sub-lethal doses of diverse drugs) a typical syndrome appears, the symptoms of which are independent of the nature of the original damaging agent and represent a response to damage of whatever cause.

Selye described various stages of the development of this syndrome, which Dr Theron Randolph soon realized were identical to the various facets he had observed in the development of allergy. The whole subject of masking, withdrawal symptomatology on avoidance of foods and the Rinkel Hyperacute Response fitted in exactly with Selye's observations in animals. The principles of adaptation and maladaptation are discussed much more extensively in Chapter 14. The concept of adaptation is dealt with quite brilliantly by Dr Randolph in his book, *Allergies: Your Hidden Enemy*, which was co-authored by Ralph Moss, and is published by Thorsons.

Fixed and cyclic food allergies

Food allergies can be divided into fixed food allergies and cyclic food allergies. A fixed food allergy is one which has probably been present since birth and will never go away. In other words, the individual may eat the food extremely rarely but will react adversely every time. He or she may avoid the food for twenty years and then still react strongly to it. These fixed food allergies are comparatively rare and certainly account for less than 5 per cent of all food allergies.

A food allergy which disappears within two years of complete avoidance of the food will generally be regarded as a cyclic food allergy. In a cyclic food allergy, the degree of reaction is related to the frequency of ingestion. One method of treatment other than desensitization (which is discussed in Chapter 10) is to avoid the food for a period of time, during which tolerance can develop. This time usually varies between two and eight months, but by definition can extend up to two years. Usually, the stronger the symptoms that the food gives, the longer it takes for tolerance to develop. Tolerance can also, in exceptional circumstances, develop within two or three weeks and this is a potent source of problems in elimination diets, which may extend over a period of abour five weeks.

Tolerance is, however, a fragile flower and can usually be maintained only if the individual eats the allergenic food every five days. If the food is consumed more frequently than this the sufferer nearly always starts to react to it again. It is, of course, vital to understand this concept. I have seen patients who identify specific food allergies on an exclusion diet. Some months later they may eat the food again by mistake but, having suffered no reaction, they conclude that their original observation was erroneous. Unless forewarned, they may then start to eat the food on a frequent basis, rapidly destroy their tolerance to it, and then start to react to it once more. These ideas about the development and subsequent maintenance of tolerance led to the development of what is known as the rotary diversified diet.

The rotary diversified diet

The rotary diversified diet is one of the major tools in this field. People with minor allergy problems or with a sensitivity to only two or three foods will rarely need to use it. Sufferers who are adequately dealt with by desensitization will not usually need to use it. Those who have a Candida problem (see Chapter 6) need it less if their Candida is treated. However, even if you do not go on to a formal rotary diet, you are advised to widen the scope of the foods you eat and to vary your diet as much as is possible. The fundamental principle of the rotary diet is that foods from specific food families are eaten only one day in every four. A typical rotary diversified diet is as followed on pages 30 and 31.

It will be seen from perusal of this diet that certain principles have been followed in devising it:

Only whole foods are included. A food mixture, for example gravy powder, contains: (1) starch – probably corn; (2) modified starch; (3) salt; (4) caramel – probably derived from glucose; (5) soya flour; (6) hydrolysed vegetable protein; (7) dried yeast; and (8) flavourings. A single product containing such a wide range of items would be inadmissible.

Food families need to be considered in devising a rotary diversified diet. The reason for this is that you can cross-react to 'relatives' of foods to which you are allergic. Foods from any food family are therefore included on the same day but excluded mostly from other days.

Another reason for considering food families is that the continual ingestion of several foods from a family can lead to the development of allergy. If garlic is eaten on Sunday, onions on Monday, asparagus on Tuesday and leeks on Wednesday, then foods are not being truly rotated. One food from this group (which is known as the LILY food family

TYPICAL ROTARY DIVERSIFIED DIET

	Day 1	Day 2	Day 3	Day 4
Protein	All red meats and their products: pork venison beef, veal, lamb milk, yogurt, all cheese	All fish: tuna, mackerel, rock salmon turbot, sole, halibut, flounder haddock, cod, perch, carp trout, salmon sardines, herring	Fowl: turkey, goose, duck chicken, pheasant, guinea fowl eggs	Shellfish: crab, shrimps, lobster clams, oysters snails, squid scallops
Vegetables	Mushrooms Sweet potatoes Squash, courgettes, pumpkin, cucumber Water chestnuts	Cabbage, broccoli, turnips, radishes, cauliflower Brussels sprouts, mustard greens, kale Lettuce, artichokes, endive Yams, yuca	Carrots, celery, parsnips, parsley All peas and beans, lentils, soya beans, alfalfa sprouts, bean sprouts (legumes) Asparagus, onions, leeks	Spinach, beetroot, Swiss chard Okra Potatoes, tomatoes, aubergine (eggplant) Peppers Corn, bamboo shoots
Fruit	Pineapple Dates Melons Peaches, apricots, nectarines, cherries, plums, prunes	Grapes, raisins Blueberries, cranberries Bananas Guavas	Strawberries, raspberries Apples, pears Rhubarb Mangoes Papayas Currants	Oranges, grapefruit, lemons, tangerines Pomegranates Figs Gooseberries Avocado

TYPICAL ROTARY DIVERSIFIED DIET

	Day 1	*Day 2*	*Day 3*	*Day 4*
Seeds and nuts	Pumpkin seeds Almonds Macadamia nuts	Sunflower seeds Pecans, walnuts	Peanuts, soy nuts Cashews, pistachios Sesame seeds	Filberts, hazelnuts, chestnuts Brazil nuts
Other	Coconut Arrowroot starch Yeast Gelatin	Tapioca Sunflower meal	Peanut butter Sesame meal Buckwheat	Olives Wheat, rye, barley, cornmeal Popcorn, cane, oats, rice, millet
Sweeteners	Whey, lactose Date sugar	Maple sugar or syrup	Honey	Molasses, malt syrup
Lard and oils	Almond oil Butter, lard, beef fat Coconut oil	Walnut oil Safflower oil, sunflower oil Any fish oils	Peanut oil, soy oil Chicken fat, turkey fat Sesame oil	Olive oil Corn oil
Herbs and spices	Nutmeg, mace Black pepper Vanilla bean	Mustard, horseradish Mint, sage, rosemary, basil, marjoram, oregano, thyme Allspice, cloves Cream of tartar	Dill, fennel, caraway, anise, chervil, cumin, coriander Ginger, cardamon, turmeric Garlic, chives	Cinnamon, bay leaf Chilli, pimiento, paprika, cayenne, red pepper
Teas	Rosehips	Blueberry Chamomile, goldenrod Mint	Papaya leaf Senna Parsley, alfalfa Sarsparilla	Juniper berry Sassafras Comfrey, hops

group) is in this case being eaten every day and this can in some cases sensitize people to the entire food group. However, the ingestion of foods from a specific food family does not need to be spaced at four-day intervals; usually, two-day intervals will be satisfactory. In other words, with the example from the LILY group, garlic and onions could be eaten on Monday, and asparagus and leeks on Wednesday, then garlic and onions again on Friday.

Many people looking at the sample rotary diversified diet will notice in it a large number of foods they have never eaten or even thought of eating in their life. In my experience, people are amazed at how much they enjoy foods they have never considered in the past. An allergy to a food is primarily linked to the frequency of ingestion of that food and so the wider and more varied the diet the better.

Obviously, if you are not being desensitized to foods, you must omit the foods to which you are allergic from this diet. In the years prior to the development of food desensitization and other developments, for example in connection with intestinal thrush, the rotary diversified diet was the only way of helping the complex multi-allergic patient. It was, however, difficult, if not impossible, for some – for example those who had to attend business lunches most of their working life. I do still encourage patients to vary their diet as much as is reasonably possible but, except in the more severe complex cases, I do not use a full rotary diversified diet. A much more comprehensive account of the rotary diet is given in such books as *Allergies: Your Hidden Enemy* by Dr T. G. Randolph and R. W. Moss, and *Coping With Your Allergies* by Natalie Golos and Francis Golos-Golbitz.

The work of Dr Richard Mackarness

In the late 1950s a British doctor, Richard Mackarness, stumbled on to the concept of food allergy. He had noted that people who lived in primitive circumstances eating primitive foods rarely became obese, and thought that obesity might result from foods such as cereals and sugars, products which had only comparatively recently been incorporated into the human diet. Whereas fruits, vegetables, meats and fish had been consumed for over 100,000 years, cereals had been consumed for only about 2,000 years, and sugar for 300 years. It was possible that mankind had not had time to adapt to these comparatively new foods. In his book *Eat Fat and Grow Slim*, against the prevailing medical wisdom of the day, he advocated a diet avoiding cereals and sugars, but allowing as much fat, protein, vegetables, and other carbohydrates as the individual required.

Many people found this diet very helpful and the book sold in enormous quantity in the UK. As a result his publishers asked him to do a lecture tour of the USA to promote the launch of the book there. At one of these lectures he met a doctor who, having listened to his lecture, said to him, 'I am sure that you are right, but possibly for the wrong reasons. Many of your patients are probably allergic to foods such as cereals and sugars. By warning them off these foods, they are probably becoming better because they are avoiding the common food allergies'. It is, of course, likely that these foods are the common food allergies because mankind has not well adapted to them.

This doctor suggested that Dr Mackarness should meet his brother-in-law, Dr Theron Randolph. Dr Mackarness responded to this idea with alacrity and became fascinated by the ideas that Dr Randolph was able to impart. When Dr Mackarness returned hom he slowly incorporated these new ideas into his day-to-day general practice. Having acquired a fair amount of experience in this field and having become entirely convinced by its validity, he then wrote *Not All in the Mind*, which was initially published in 1976. In 1980 he followed this success with his next book, *Chemical Victims*. With these two books he succeeded in opening up awareness of this subject.

Spreading the word

Although the medical profession as a whole was not interested in food and chemical allergy, a small group of doctors, of which I was one, had their curiosity aroused. In 1979, about 19 doctors formed the British Clinical Ecology Group. By January 1982 the number had swelled to over 100 and the group changed and became the British Society for Clinical Ecology. Various clinical trials began to be published, substantiating the claim that food allergy was a very important factor in human disease, including arthritis.

In 1978, Dr Ronald Finn wrote a paper entitled 'Food Allergy, Fact or Fiction?', published in *The Lancet*, describing a trial which demonstrated that food allergy was the major factor in a series of patients who had, among other symptoms, a history of palpitations. The trial was a double-blind trial where patients were fed foods that were suspected to be allergens in situations where they did not know what they were eating. For example, the foods were introduced via a stomach tube. This trial was reported widely in the media and prompted more letters to *The Lancet* than any other trial in the previous few years.

In May 1979, Dr Ellen Grant had her trial on migraine and food allergy also published in *The Lancet*, showing that 85 per cent of sufferers could become headache-free if they avoided foods to which they had been found to be sensitive. A further trial on the same subject with similar results was published by Dr Jonathan Brostoff and Dr Jean Monro in *The Lancet* in July 1980.

In November 1982, Dr John Hunter and his colleagues at Addenbrooke's Hospital in Cambridge produced a paper on food intolerance and the irritable bowel syndrome. In this paper, again published in *The Lancet*, they demonstrated that two-thirds of patients with this condition could lose their symptoms if they avoided specific foods to which they had been found sensitive. As with all allergy problems, the foods involved varied quite widely and a number of double-blind studies were completed.

October 1983 saw the publication of Professor Soothill's trial of migraine and food allergy in children. The trial was performed at Great Ormond Street and was undoubtedly the most comprehensive trial done on this subject. In many people's view it substantiated the view that migraine was a food allergy problem in a very high proportion of patients. In 1984 Dr Pamela Graham and some co-workers at Brighton General Hospital published a paper demonstrating that food allergy was a major cause of eczema in children in the *British Journal of Dermatology*.

In 1982 Dr Gail Darlington and I read a paper before the Heberden Society on food allergy and rheumatoid arthritis. In this trial we demonstrated that about 65 per cent of patients with rheumatoid arthritis responded well to an elimination diet. This small trial encouraged us to go on to the more elaborate placebo-controlled trial which was published in *The Lancet* in 1986. The details of this trial are in Chapter 12.

Dr Theron Randolph extensively reported his work on rheumatoid arthritis in the book *Clinical Ecology*, published by Charles C. Thomas in Springfield, Illinois, and edited by Lawrence Dickey.

In 1980 there was the trial on 22 patients with rheumatoid

arthritis published in *Clinical Allergy*. The authors of this trial were Dr Len McEwan and Dr A. J. Hicklin. The summer and autumn of 1984 saw the publication of the large American trial of rheumatoid arthritis and allergy, which was published in the journal *Clinical Ecology*. This trial was carried out at three separate environmental control units run respectively by Dr T. Randolph, Dr W. J. Rea and Dr R. A.Carroll. These trials are all reported in detail in Chapter 12.

Large international meetings of the British and American Societies for Clinical Ecology were held at Torquay in 1984 and at Harrogate in 1987. At these meetings, which were attended by nearly 300 doctors, papers were read by physicians from different parts of the world reporting studies of food and chemical sensitivity in relation to a number of diseases, such as hyperactivity in children, recurrent ear infections in children, rheumatoid arthritis, and recurrent thrombophlebitis.

In 1987 the British Society for Clinical Ecology had attracted a considerable number of consultant physicians to its ranks. Because the word 'ecology' had the flavour of some political groupings we changed the name of the society to the British Society for Allergy and Environmental Medicine in deference to their wishes. The society in America changed its name to the American Academy of Environmental Medicine.

The concept that food allergy is an important factor in disease has therefore advanced enormously in the past few years and more and more physicians from academic medicine are becoming actively involved in it. However, the subject is somewhat bedevilled by controversies over different methods of testing and it is perhaps appropriate at this point to discuss and comment on these various methods.

Allergy tests

1. Elimination tests

Elimination diets are undoubtedly the 'bench-mark' against which all other methods of testing should be measured. When going through an elimination diet the individual sees in real life what is happening. If you have severe arthritis and then limit your diet to a handful of safe foods for a few days and your symptoms disappear, you know where you stand. It is also not a great sacrifice when a few days can change your whole future outlook from unmitigated pessimism to great optimism. The test also has the virtue that it is both simple and inexpensive. If improvement is not attained then food allergy can be excluded.

The subsequent phase of reintroducing foods into your diet may also be simple, but it is fair to say that in someone with a large number of sensitivities it can be very complicated.

This approach is used, mostly for other conditions, in National Health hospitals and has developed a fair degree of respectability over the past decade. I have devoted the whole of Chapter 9 to this subject later in the book.

2. Intradermal provocative skin-testing and neutralization

This is a vast improvement and refinement on standard skin prick-testing which has been used for many years in hospitals. There have been about nine clinical trials which have established its validity and used competently it is a vital and extremely useful method of both diagnosis and treatment. About 15 clinics in the UK use the test extensively, and in the USA it is used currently by over 400 clinics. Without it we would not be able to help a large proportion of our more complicated patients. The test and concept is so important that I have devoted two later chapters (10 and 11) to the uses of this method and one chapter (13) to the trials validating its usage.

3. Prick testing

This is a fairly useful test for inhalant allergies but does not really help in the diagnosis of food allergy. It is this simple fact which has, in my opinion, held back until recently the development of interest in food allergy.

The test involves placing a single drop of allergen extract on the inner forearm. A lancet is introduced through the drop of extract on the skin at an acute angle and, having slightly penetrated the skin, is given a deliberate vertical lift before being removed. Responses to these tests are read after 10-20 minutes. Many of the tests can be performed within a few minutes of each other and the whole test is therefore both simple and quick to perform. Unhappily, it is not very effective because most patients with well-established food allergies will fail to react positively to this test. As we have become familiar with the intradermal provocative neutralizing test it has become apparent why prick tests are so useful for diagnosing inhalant allergies but useless for diagnosing food allergies. I have detailed these thoughts in Chapters 10 and 11.

Because prick tests have been used for so long, many people, including physicians, place unwarranted credence on their results. I have known patients with genuine food allergies who have been informed categorically that their allergies do not exist, purely on the basis of this test which can therefore do more harm than good. Dr Keith Eaton of Reading has recently published a trial showing that the prick test is of no value in diagnosing food allergy. As he put it, one is better off spinning a coin to determine food allergies than relying on this test.

4. The RAST Test (Radioallergosorbent Test)

This test involves taking a blood sample and measuring the quantity of immunoglobulin E antibodies that form when this blood is exposed to different allergens. It is thought that the higher the count of IgE antibodies, the more allergic the patient. The RAST test is fairly useful in diagnosing allergies to dust, dust mite, moulds, animal danders, pollens, and some foods. It has, however, many drawbacks: (a) it can only be used for testing a very limited number of food allergies; (b) it costs about five times more per allergy tested than does provocative neutralization testing; (c) it measures only immediate responses, and many food-allergic reactions are delayed; (d) RAST tests take a few days before results are available – provocative neutralization skin testing results are available almost immediately; (e) interpretation and technique vary somewhat from laboratory to laboratory, and false negatives and false positives often occur; (f) it is quite probable that in the future the RAST test may be refined and become more useful. However, at its best, even if this does happen, the only therapeutic approach that will stem from it would be dietary avoidance of the incriminated foods with all its attendant difficulties and disadvantages. Comparative tests done in the United States between RAST and provocative intradermal neutralization have shown that the provocative neutralization testing is superior and of course it has the inestimable advantage of enabling you to eat the foods to which you are sensitive.

5. Cytotoxic testing

This is just about the most controversial of all tests for food allergy. There are a few physicians who enthusiastically promote cytotoxic testing, but the whole of the conventional allergy estabishment and most members of the British Society for Allergy and Environmental Medicine are very sceptical about its value. It does, of course, have the superficial attraction of suggesting that countless food and chemical allergies can be diagnosed from a single sample of intravenous blood. The term cytotoxic literally means 'having a toxic effect on cells'.

The blood sample is incubated on a microscope slide with a weak solution of suspected food allergen and the effect on certain specific white cells is noted. In a positive test the polymorph leucocytes (one type of white cell) slow down, become rounded and, in strongly positive cases, disintegrate. There is no doubt that this phenomenon occurs, but the interpretation of the results depends on the varying judgements of different technicians.

Currently an automated version of this test is being assessed in the Immunology Department of a major London teaching hospital. By using the automated technique one can exclude the individual human error. Initial assessment of the automated technique gives some grounds for optimism. Certainly, if this became a reliable test, it could be extesively used by practitioners with little knowledge of allergy and this would doubtless lead to a wider application of these principles in general medical management.

The biggest criticism of the cytotoxic test as it is currently used, and in my opinion a fair one, is that companies offering the test often do so directly to the public. Sometimes they appear to discover huge numbers of food sensitivities and as a result some people may end up on a very harsh and possibly nutritionally inadequate diet, unsupervised by anyone with any knowledge of nutrition. Of course, such a situation arises partly because many physicians in the National Health Service stubbornly refuse to have any involvement with this field at all.

6. Applied Kinesiology

This method is particularly favoured by chiropractors, some of whom have taken an interest in the field of food allergy. Initially the practitioner establishes the patient's muscle strength and tone by observing how easily he or she can lift, for example, a 50lb (23kg) weight. An allergen is introduced, usually under the tongue, and the muscle tone again measured. The theory is that an allergic reaction will weaken the muscle tone and this can be detected by the practitioner. There may be something in this test, but there has been absolutely no scientific validation of it as yet. At the moment, as there are relatively well-validated alternatives in existence, I feel that these approaches should be used in preference to applied kinesiology.

7. Radionics

Several people in the United Kingdom claim to be able to diagnose food allergies from hair samples. A pendulum is dangled over the hair sample, and if it rotates in one way allergy is indicated, if it rotates the opposite way it is not. Although I accept that there are several very strange magnetic phenomena which we do not yet understand, this particular test stretches credibility to breaking point. I have had many patients who have seen me after they have been tested in this way and the allergies that we have detected have borne little relationship to their hair test results.

The worst aspect of fringe tests, such as cytotoxic testing, kinesiology and radionics, is that many physicians who find dubious the concept of food sensitivity have seized upon these tests and their complete lack of scientific validation to criticize serious allergists who, in fact, do not use these tests anyway.

8. Sublingual testing

When I was first interested in the subject of food allergy I did quite a lot of tests using this method. The principle is the same as the intradermal provocative test. Solutions are made up in nine separate concentrations with a 1 in 5 dilution factor between one strength and the next. The first strength is the strongest, the second is one-fifth weaker and so on.

The technique consists of placing one measured drop of the food to be tested under the patient's tongue using a specially-designed dropper pipette. The area under the tongue is one of great absorbability as the large sublingual veins are present there. The patient lies quietly on a couch and any resulting symptoms are noted. It is also usual to take the pulse and record the size of the pupils at intervals. If symptoms or other changes occur, successively weaker levels are administered until they are counteracted. A more elaborate description of this technique can be found in Richard Mackarness' book *Not All in the Mind*

(Pan Books, 1976).

Sometimes, particularly with very soluble foodstuffs such as milk, tea, coffee, orange, etc., one can see dramatic and obvious reactions when these are introduced under the tongue. With less soluble items, particularly items such as wheat and corn, reactions can easily fail to materialize despite the fact that the individual has a wheat or corn sensitivity, and I cannot recall seeing anyone middle-aged who has had a dramatic reaction to wheat, corn, or any other cereal given sublingually.

The other disadvantage is that it is much more difficult to obtain the neutralizing level when foods are tested in this way. This form of testing is inferior to intradermal provocation testing, as intradermal provocation testing has two pillars on which the assessment can be made. One pillar represents the symptoms which are being induced or relieved. The other pillar is the appearance of the wheal. These two facets complement each other and the wheal changes normally correlate with the changes in symptom pattern. Some people, however, with allergies identified as a result of the elimination diet, the sublingual testing, or even the intradermal testing, will fail to induce any symptoms whatsoever. With the intradermal testing one at least can observe the wheal response, but with sublingual testing one just has to record the test as negative, although earlier testing has proved that there was a positive reaction.

Treatments for food allergies

There is one fairly well-established form of treatment for food allergy, which is the **provocative intradermal neutralization** treatment, given either by injection or sublingual drops and validated by the trials mentioned in Chapter 10.

Rather less well validated is **enzyme potentiated desensitization** developed by Dr Len McEwen, who used to work at the Department of Allergy at St Mary's Hospital, Paddington. In this type of desensitization a large number of allergens in a container are strapped on to an area of scarified skin on the arm. Dr McEwen does not claim that the technique works immediately as it does with neutralization therapy, but claims good responses over a period of months. He has published details of a trial in the journal *Clinical Ecology* showing the approach to be of distinct value in the management of ulcerative colitis. Presumably if it works in ulcerative colitis it should work in other conditions related to food allergy. Dr McEwen is an extremely capable physician and he now has several other physicians following his lead in this area.

The next two techniques have much less validity but are included to complete this review.

(a) Auto-immune urine therapy

This therapy was originally introduced in 1947 and has a small number of enthusiastic advocates. The technique consists of collecting a urine sample the morning after you have eaten a meal containing all the items to which you suspect or know that you are sensitive. The urine is filtered through micropore filters and is injected in specific and increasing quantities, into your thigh. A variation on this technique is to be titrated to your own urine intradermally and to find a neutralizing level in the same way as is done with foods. The neutralizing dose can then either be taken by injection or sublingual drops.

This treatment has a valid immunological basis as many antigens are excreted in the urine. By subsequently reintroducing them into the body it is possible to build up the level of T-lymphocytes, which is the best single indicator of the competence of the immune system. However, antigens from the kidneys are also being re-injected and this can cause the immune system to start repelling its own tissues. As this can be very damaging to the kidneys, auto-immune urine injection therapy is a procedure to be avoided.

(b) Acupuncture

This ancient Chinese healing art claims to be able to heal an enormous variety of mental and physical ailments. The theory is that the body's energy passes along imaginary lines called meridians. These meridians supposedly connect sensitive areas under the skin with diseased internal organs, which are often situated a long way away from the specific skin sites. The meridian lines are not explainable by any Western knowledge of anatomy or physiology. The treatment entails inserting long thin needles into the specific sensitive areas. The needles remain in situ for about 20 or 30 minutes and there is some variation in the way in which the needles are used. Sometimes they are twirled, sometimes wired to electrical currents, and sometimes pre-heated.

Recent work completed in Scotland has shown that stimulating certain parts of the body also stimulates the pituitary gland in the brain. This in turn can produce chemicals called endorphins. These chemicals resemble various narcotics in their effect and can relieve pain and produce a general sense of well-being. It may well be this effect which accounts for the benefit that many patients find with acupuncture.

These, therefore, are exciting times for physicians involved in testing for food sensitivity. Certainly a cheap, easy, practical method for diagnosing food sensitivies would be a great boon. Personally, I think a judicious combination of elimination diets and intradermal provocative testing gives very reasonable answers and sorts out the problems in most patients.

3 Chemical sensitivity and arthritis

After food allergy, chemical sensitivity appears to be the next most important factor in the causation of arthritic symptoms. The problem can be subdivided into: (a) chemicals which we inhale; and (b) chemicals which we eat. The man who discovered and then developed the concept of chemical sensitivity was Dr Theron Randolph of Chicago, Illinois. Dr Randolph had observed enormous improvement occurring in many patients with arthritis of varying types as a result of food elimination and challenge followed by avoidance of test-positive foods. However, there was a proportion of people who only partially improved or did not improve at all.

In 1947 he was consulted by a patient who had been generally regarded by her medical advisers to be a hypochondriac. As a child she had had several classical allergic problems, such as hives and an allergic runny nose, but these left her as she grew up. Later in life she developed extremely severe headaches, severe fatigue, tension, and asthma. She noticed that whenever she drove through heavily polluted parts of Chicago or found herself behind a diesel lorry, she would become very ill and sometimes virtually unconscious. On several occasions she almost crashed her car, only to be saved at the last minute by her passenger.

She also noted that she felt particularly ill when she visited her pine cabin in the woods which she often used for holidays. Dr Randolph tested various samples from this cabin and it turned out that the pine itself was the main culprit. Later she noticed that gas from her gas cooker and odours from rubber mattresses, soft plastics, etc. all produced adverse responses.

Eventually this picture fitted into a pattern when she consulted Dr Randolph on a day that a major storm was threatening the Chicago area. All the other patients had cancelled their appointments for the afternoon and Dr Randolph was able to review 50 pages of typewritten observations of what appeared to be making this patient ill. He suddenly realized that virtually all her problems were related to the time of specific exposure to petrochemicals or man-made chemicals derived from petroleum. Even the reactivity to pine fitted into the picture as oil and gas are ultimately derived from the decomposition of huge primeval pine forests over a period of millions of years crushed beneath rock strata. Pine trees, incidentally, give off an odour called turpenes which, when combined with low oxygen in the atmosphere, tend to lead to a condition called 'mountain madness' in susceptible individuals. Later it was discovered that this patient also reacted to ingested chemicals, such as artificial food colourants, the phenolic resin lining of tinned food cans, and food sprayed with insecticides, which of course are derived from petroleum.

Once this break-through had occurred it soon became obvious that this patient was not unique. Other patients with seemingly incomprehensible disease patterns began to fall into a distinct group. As more cases were seen, it emerged that the most important pollutants were household gas, formaldehyde, and the pesticides found in the food supplies.

It is not surprising that some human beings should have some problems with chemicals. Living organisms can adapt to many changes in their environment, but this adaptation often takes many generations and tends not to be universal. Since the Second World War in particular there has been an enormous explosion in newly discovered chemicals, and the chemical industry has now quite revolutionized modern life. In Europe and the USA hundreds of billions of pounds of chemicals are produced annually and over 25,000 different chemicals are in common use in the UK alone. Many of these chemicals find their ways into our bodies.

The testing of chemicals is hardly comprehensive and certainly takes no account of people who may be highly susceptible. As yet, no one has any idea of the cumulative effect of all these chemicals and this is the most worrying aspect of the whole problem. Nobody knows how these individual chemicals interreact within the confines of the human frame. The twentieth century has been rightly described as an enormous, uncontrolled experiment on the human race.

How then can chemical sensitivities relate to the patient who has joint pain, swelling and stiffness? I propose firstly to describe some of the problems encountered and then to explain how to isolate them.

Chemicals that are inhaled

Inhaled chemical problems can be roughly divided into indoor air pollution and outdoor air pollution, and many people may be surprised to learn that indoor air pollution is generally more of a problem. Outdoor air pollution, which is well known because of such phenomena as smog and traffic fumes, is usually only intermittent and often very obvious. The effects of indoor air pollution, by contrast, are usually more continuous, more hidden, more subtle, and more significant. Many hydrocarbon-sensitive people are aware of the fact that intermittently present hydrocarbons such as perfumes, petrol fumes, nail varnish, printer's ink, and dry cleaning fluids are able to induce symptoms of one sort or another, but these individuals are virtually always ignorant of the fact that their domestic gas or oil is playing a part in their problems. The combustion products of the burning of these fuels within the confines of the house linger in the house for days, even after the utilities are turned off.

Because of its relative cheapness, natural gas is now present in a very high proportion of British homes, both for central heating and for cooking. Gas is more commonly implicated in arthritis than any other single chemical. Sponge rubber in upholstery, mattresses, cushions and so forth can cause problems with some individuals. As with plastics, the effects tend to be very insidious. More obvious pollutants, such as cigarette, pipe or cigar smoke, can upset certain patients with arthritis, either by obviously increasing arthritis symptoms (this occurs only rarely) or inducing other symptoms, such as headache, fatigue, nausea, or cough.

Outdoor air pollution plays only a small part in the arthritis story. Certainly adverse reactions of any type to pollutants such as petrol fumes, diesel fumes and so forth should raise the possibility in the allergist's mind that more insidious reactions to continuous indoor pollutants may also be present.

Chemicals in food

Multiple fruit sensitivity

The earliest recognized case of a specific chemical sensitivity was that of a man who reported severe headaches whenever he ate apples. He discovered one day that when he ate apples from an old orchard which had not been sprayed for many years, there was no adverse effect. Dr Randolph, whose patient this was, later fed him on a double-blind basis several apples, some of which had been sprayed and some not. The man consistently reacted only to the sprayed items. Suddenly, an explanation was at hand for cases of multiple fruit sensitivity.

All the early allergists had noted that many patients claimed they reacted to nearly all fruits, which was surprising as they came from so many dissociated food families. Most of these patients were not, in fact, reacting to the fruits themselves, but to the spray residues on them. These sprays permeate the whole fruit and peeling the fruit rarely helps. Anyone with multiple fruit sensitivities should therefore obtain a sample of organically-grown fruit to see if the organically-grown item has the same adverse effect as the commercially-produced item.

Sometimes patients report multiple *vegetable* sensitivities and these can also turn out to be chemical susceptibility problems. Leafy vegetables such as cabbage, broccoli, Brussels sprouts, cauliflower, lettuce, and spinach are particularly liable to be sprayed and many people react to this whole range.

Common chemical additives

Chlorinated hydrocarbons are also used to spray the feed of many animals and these chemicals can contaminate the fat, particularly of animals such as beef, lamb, and poultry. As the hydrocarbons are mostly located in the fat, removing the fat from these animals can often reduce or eliminate the problem.

Bananas are normally ripened by exposure to ethylene gas. They are still green when they arrive from the exporting country as they travel well like this. A few hours' exposure to ethylene gas makes them yellow, and a high proportion of patients with hydrocarbon sensitivity react to these bananas but find non-gassed bananas cause no problems. In a similar way, some people who apparently react adversely to coffee are in reality not reacting to coffee itself, but to the fact that most coffee is roasted over a gas flame.

Sulphur dioxide is another chemical which can cause problems. People are frequently puzzled as to why they react to French-fried potatoes prepared in a restaurant but not to those eaten at home. Almost all restaurants buy pre-cut and packed

French-fried potatoes and they are soaked in sulphur dioxide to stop them browning at the edges. In another example, some of my patients who were apparently reacting to corn turned out to be in reality reacting to sulphur dioxide. Prior to processing, the corn kernel is soaked in sulphur dioxide solution in order to prevent the corn fermenting.

Cucumbers, apples, and green peppers are foods which are frequently coated with paraffin wax to improve their appearance and keep them edible for longer periods of time. This paraffin wax is derived from petroleum and can therefore cause problems similar to those mentioned earlier.

Coming loosely under the category of chemicals in food is the subject of chemicals occurring in our tap water. The most common problem by far is chlorine, which is of course added to tap water in order to curtail the spread of infection. In this context it is very effective, but nevertheless quite a large number of chemically-sensitive individuals react adversely to it. Tony G., whose case history appears in Chapter 1, reacted very convincingly to chlorine and this proved to be one of the major factors causing his osteoarthritis. It is for this reason that when I place patients on a low-risk allergy diet, I encourage them to use bottled spring water to start with.

Most people with chlorine sensitivity can tolerate tap water which has been boiled for eight minutes. Chlorine is volatile and boiling will normally remove it. There are chlorine filters on the market which remove enough chlorine for most people to tolerate the filtered tap water.

Insecticide sprays, if used in large quantities, can permeate through the soil, washed down by rain water, and can therefore contaminate the underground water tables. Those who are exquisitely sensitive to these insecticides may find it difficult to find a water supply that they can tolerate, as the insecticides are virtually impossible to remove. These patients sometimes have to drink spring water collected from underground tables in mountain areas. This is a comparatively rare problem for arthritic sufferers in Great Britain, but in the USA, where crop spraying is practised on a much larger scale, it is becoming an extremely difficult problem for some people.

Food colourants have received a lot of publicity, particularly in connection with hyperactivity. The Feingold diet, which eliminates all colourants and other additives from food, has been used extensively in dealing with this condition, although it is now known that the additives are only part of the overall problem. Items such as coloured ice creams, confectionery, and soft drinks such as colas are well-known to contain such dyes. What surprises many people is that butters and margarines often contain dyes to make them look more yellow.

I have touched only briefly on this subject, which is now becoming a huge subject in itself. It is covered in much greater detail in Dr Theron Randolph's book *Human Ecology and Susceptibility to the Chemical Environment*, which was the first book produced on this subject. There is also extensive coverage in the book *Allergies: Your Hidden Enemy*, again by Dr Randolph, but written in collaboration with R. W. Moss Ph.D.Dr Richard Mackarness devoted a whole book to the subject and called it *Chemical Victims*.

Diagnosing the problem

Many readers may wonder at this point how a physician can possibly sort out all the possibilities on an out-patient basis – and in some patients it can certainly be very difficult. The history, as has been pointed out, can usually excite the allergist's suspicions. Intradermal provocative skin testing with synthetic ethanol, natural gas extracts, formaldehyde, phenol, etc. can further heighten the suspicions and then temporary avoidance can ultimately confirm the matter. There are whole chapters on intradermal skin testing later in this book (Chapters 10-11), as applied to food and chemicals. Suffice it to say at this point that if someone has a positive skin reaction to synthetic ethanol, chemical sensitivity is likely to be very important.

Synthetic ethanol is a liquid condensate of ethylene gas which is an extremely typical hydrocarbon and present in most petrochemicals, including gas. If the positive skin reaction is accompanied by symptoms on the top strength of synthetic ethanol, suspicion mounts to a virtual certainty, particularly if the symptoms are then relieved by finding a weaker 'neutralizing' dose which turns off the symptoms. If symptoms of arthritis can be 'turned on' by one concentration of a chemical and 'turned off' by another, this is very persuasive evidence that the chemical is relevant to that patient's problems (see Chapter 11).

If skin-test positives are found to items such as synthetic ethanol, gas, formaldehyde, or phenol, these items should be avoided when the arthritis sufferer goes on to the elimination diet.

Hydrocarbon sensitivity never exists by itself, in my experience. If it does exist, then it is vital that someone undergoing the diet as an out-patient should do so in an environment which avoids the chemical sensitivities that have been identified. This often means just turning off the gas at the mains and ventilating the house before the diet commences. If formaldehyde or phenol are involved it may be impossible to remove these from the house temporarily, or it may be necessary to stay elsewhere while on the diet. If chemical sensitivities are known to be present, only organic items should be used in the initial low-risk diet. Furthermore, when symptoms have cleared and foods are being reintroduced, organic foods only should still be used until a good basic diet of 'compatible' foods has been obtained. When we have got to this point, chemically contaminated foods can then be tried. Often the reaction to chemically contaminated food can be very insidious and build up over a week or so, and this is the reason why chemically contaminated foods are not tested from the very beginning.

The environmental control unit

Admission into a good environmental control unit is the ultimate strategy for sorting out arthritis which fails to respond to out-patient management. Sometimes an arthritic condition is too complex to respond to the sort of measures I have outlined.It is unusual for someone with rheumatoid or non-specific arthritis to enter an environmental control unit, fast for five or six days, and still have the main symptoms of arthritis.

The few that do not improve in such circumstances are probably those whose whole immune system and ability to recover have been damaged by many years of treatment with Cortisone or its derivatives. Sometimes other powerful disease-modifying drugs (such as Gold or Penicillamine), if given long enough and in high enough dosage, might have the same adverse effect. In addition there are a few people whose arthritic symptoms appear to be linked with intestinal candidiasis or gut parasites. Of course these people take the flora of their gut into the environmental unit with them and so they will remain ill, despite all the other precautions.

In the UK at the time of writing there are two environmental control units: The Airedale Allergy Centre in Keighley in Yorkshire, which is run by Dr Jonathon Maberly; and Breakspeare Hospital in King's Langley, Hertfordshire, an allergy and environmental medicine hospital run by Dr Jean Monro. In the

USA there are several such units. The two best-known are the one in Chicago run by Dr Theron Randolph, and the Environmental Health Centre in Dallas, run by Dr William Rea. Dr Rea has recently been appointed Professor of Environmental Medicine at the prestigious Robens Institute of Toxicology at the University of Surrey in England. He is the first physician in the world to hold a Professorial Chair in this subject.

The environmental control unit represents in my opinion the most scientific approach in clinical medicine to the causation of many disease processes. The crux of such a programme is:

the concurrent avoidance of multiple inhaled and ingested excitants over a period of a few days, during which time chronic symptoms usually disappear

the subsequent reintroduction of foods or inhalants one at a time and the observation of any adverse response to these items.

Ideally, an environmental unit should be purpose-built and situated in an area of low pollution, such as in the countryside. Materials used in the construction of the building should be hard and not prone to out-gas. Bricks, concrete, metal, and wood (other than pine) are satisfactory. Walls are ideally clad with materials such as ceramic tiles or porcelainized steel. Flooring should consist of marble or terrazzo tiles embedded in concrete rather than stuck with adhesives. Hard wood stained with polyurethane varnish or vinyl tiles are not quite so satisfactory. Interior decoration and furnishing should use items such as cotton, leather, felt, natural fabrics, metal, and wood (not pine). Heating can be supplied by electricity or by hot water radiators as long as the central heating boiler (if gas) is situated outside the unit itself.

Personnel working in the unit and visitors should not wear perfumes or after-shave and of course should not smoke. Recently dry-cleaned suits can pose a problem and ideally they should be changed outside the unit to cotton clothing rather like that worn in operating theatres.

Items not welcome in such units would include: (1) sponge rubber in mattresses, chairs or carpet underlays; (2) soft plastic covers, curtains or suitcases, or plasticized bed linen or furniture surfaces; (3) plaster board or fabrics treated with formaldehyde.

I have spent time in both the major American environmental

control units that have been mentioned. One has the feeling of observing the medicine of the future in its most advanced form. I saw patient after patient fasted in these clean environments with severe forms of arthritis very evident at the beginning of the fast. By the fifth or sixth day they had virtually all cleared their symptoms. What was impressive was that it was all so routine to the staff as they had been seen these miracles so many times and so constantly they were no longer impressed with them.

After symptom clearance patients are challenged first with organic foods and later with inhaled items. The inhalant tests are done in 'sniff boxes' which are rather like telephone booths. Patients are exposed to chemicals in these booths while under observation. They do not know the precise nature of the chemicals to which they are being exposed, but later the results of these tests are discussed with them. People with certain chemical sensitivities, such as gas, may have to make engineering changes to their homes. Some have to take neutralizing drops or injection, and some may have to live off organic food and bottled spring waters. Those in the latter category have the hardest time, but often they are amongst the severest sufferers. Talking to them, I had no doubt that they preferred their slightly restricted lifestyle to a lifetime of joint pains, swelling, and interminable drugs.

4 Alcohol and smoking in relation to arthritis

Alcohol

Very large numbers of arthritis sufferers notice that the consumption of certain alcoholic beverages will almost invaribly led to a major flare-up of their arthritic symptoms. This is a very positive indicator that food allergy is important in the causation of those individual's problems,

In the late 1940s, Dr Theron Randolph made a considerable intuitive leap in realizing that reactions to alcoholic beverages were caused by reactions to the constituents of these beverages and not to the alcohol itself. What made the reactions to these beverages so obvious is the rapid absorption of their constituents. Everyone is familiar with the very rapidly observable effect of, for example, four double Scotches consumed in quick succession. The main constituent of Scotch whisky is grain which when consumed normally (e.g. in the form of bread) takes many hours to be absorbed in any quantity. In the form of Scotch whisky it is absorbed in a few minutes. Part of the reason for this rapid absorption is that, whereas food is normally absorbed only in the intestines, alcohol is absorbed throughout the intestinal tract, starting from the mouth, going through the stomach and duodenum, into the intestines. Dr Randolph coined the phrase that reactions to alcoholic beverages represent 'food allergy in a jet-propelled vehicle'.

Most of the main alcoholic beverages are derived from foods such as wheat, corn, cane sugar, yeast, grapes, and potatoes. These items represent the more common food allergens. Remembering the concept of masking, it is obvious that to a wheat-allergic person a dose of an alcoholic beverage containing wheat will have a quicker masking effect than wheat eaten conventionally because of the rapid absorptive effect. Hence, if allergy to wheat can lead to addiction to wheat, addiction to whisky will follow if the drinker is not careful. Alcoholism has been termed the acme of food allergy and there is no doubt in my mind, having dealt with a number of alcoholics, that this is true. Sometimes, however, the rapidity of the absorption of the alcoholic beverage is such that it 'breaks through the masking process' and can give the patient a direct reaction to the food rather than a masking effect.

Conversely, if the alcoholic beverage contains a substance, for example grapes or a resin or a preserving chemical, which is not regularly present in the drinker's diet, then there may well be an unmasked hyperacute reaction, made even more acute by the rapidity of absorption.

Alcoholism and food allergy

The fact that alcoholism and food allergy are inextricably interwoven is of course important to arthritic people who are addicted to alcohol. In most cases they are allergic/addicted to the common constituents of alcoholic beverages, such as cereals, sugar, and yeast, and this allergy/addiction can only be eradicated if the foodstuff is concurrently removed from both diet and drinking habits. Because of the widespread ignorance of this concept, alcoholics usually continue to eat the foods to which they are allergic while trying to avoid them in the form of alcoholic beverages. The dried-out alcoholic is therefore deprived of the quickest and most effective 'masking shot'. Most feel tense or depressed or headachy, and the desire for alcohol often remains extremely strong for many years.

It follows from this that some alcoholics in whom specific allergies have been identified can, as long as they modify their drinking habits, consume certain alcoholic beverages without suffering a reaction. This ingestion, though, has to be done with some caution as there is a chance that they will develop a sensitivity to another food if they have a tendency to food sensitivities in any case. If this new food is consumed frequently in this very potent form, i.e. alcohol, it is quite possible that new sensitivities will arise, and so such consumption should be limited to occasional social events.

The exception to all of this is, of course, someone who has a yeast sensitivity, as yeast is present in all alcoholic beverages. As yet, there has been no large published study in which the interrelationship of alcohol and food allergy has been investigated. There have, however, been numerous individual case reports, particularly from Dr Theron Randolph, Dr Marshall Mandell and Dr Richard Mackarness, and their observations have all supported this view.

I have seen many remarkable results when adopting this approach and one patient particularly sticks in my mind. I was consulted by Mr W. K., aged 44, a 'dried-out' alcoholic. The beverage to which he had been addicted was vodka, and since ceasing to drink it he had remained extremely tense, necessitating the ingestion of approximately 60mg of Valium each day. He also suffered from numerous headaches and he told me that he felt he was on the verge of returning to his drinking habits. After six days on a low-risk allergy diet he felt immensely improved and discovered he no longer needed to take Valium. He reintroduced foods to his diet in a similar way to that described in Chapter 9. He was fine until he tried potato (a major constituent of most vodkas) and the ingestion of this food reproduced all his old symptoms. At the time of this reaction I had immense difficulty in persuading him to keep to his diet and to keep off a vodka binge. He managed to follow my advice and the reaction wore off in a couple of days. Subsequently, avoiding potatoes, he had no need to take any more Valium, had no tension, no headaches and no desire to start drinking again.

The law does not require that the contents of alcoholic beverages be stated on the bottle and in general they are allowed to remain a trade secret. However, as a result of discussions with representatives of some major alcohol manufacturers, it is possible to put together a rough guide to the content of the major alcoholic beverages obtainable in this country. Most of the information presented below relates predominantly to products from the Distillers Corporation, who are the major suppliers of alcholic beverages in Britain. Vodkas, for example, can be made from a very wide range of foods and the vodka cited in this example is made by Smirnoff. Much of the information presented here was subsequently verified by patients with known food sensitivies who have managed to observe which alcoholic beverages they can tolerate and which they cannot. There follows a breakdown of the most commonly consumed alcoholic beverages.

It must be added that wines may contain a number of chemicals which are not mentioned in this list. The cheaper wines, particularly those imported in bulk, will normally have chemicals added to them to stop them deteriorating

Always present = \ Sometimes present = O	Corn	Wheat, Barley, Rye	Oats	Rice	Potatoes	Grapes	Plum	Citrus	Cherry	Apples	Hops	Juniper	Cinnamon	Mint	Miscellaneous Herbs	Cactus	Beet Sugar	Cane Sugar
Blended Scotch Whisky	\	\															O	O
Malt Scotch Whisky	O	\															O	O
Canadian Blended Whisky	\	\				\	\	O									O	\
Irish Whisky		\	\															O
Blended Irish Whisky	\	\				\	\	O								O	O	
Gin (Grain)	\	\	O	O					\			\	O	O	\		O	O
Gin (Cane) High & Dry												\	\	\	\			\
Vodka					O												\	\
Jamaican Rum																		\
Tequila																\		\
Beer	\	\	O	\							\							
Grape Brandy	O					\											O	O
Cordials & Liqueurs	\	\	O	O	O	\	\	\	\			\	\	\			\	\
Grape Wine	O					\											\	\
Sherry	\					\											\	\
Champagne						\										\		
Cider	\									\							\	\
Vermouth	O	O	O			\											\	\
Cognac						\											O	O
Cherry Brandy	O								\								O	O

Please note that yeast occurs in all alcoholic beverages.

while travelling. As most travellers know, cheap wines do not travel well in the normal course of events and preserving chemicals have to be added to maintain them in good condition. Reaction to these chemicals is extremely prevalent and accounts I think for the common observation that cheap wine can cause a nasty hangover, whereas more expensive wine does not. The severe hangover which some people may experience with certain alcoholic beverages is usually due in my opinion to specific food sensitivities occuring in those particular beverages. A more comprehensive review of this subject is given by Dr Theron G. Randolph in the book entitled *Clinical Ecology*, published in 1976 by Charles C. Thomas.

Smoking

Smoking, and particularly cigarette smoking, has a major effect on the production of arthritis in some patients.

It is interesting to speculate what it is about cigarettes or other forms of smoking that causes these problems with arthritic sufferers. As with all items that are ingested or inhaled on a frequent basis, it is possible that human beings can become sensitized and, as allergies seem to be linked with frequent exposure, it is not surprising that some people can become sensitive to something they are exposed to maybe twenty to forty times a day. Often, after testing, patients appear to have reacted to the whole of the *Solanaceae* food family. This food family contains tobacco, potatoes, tomatoes, peppers, aubergine (eggplant), etc. The cigarette smoking has probably sensitized them to all these foods. Tobacco may cross-react with and therefore cross-mask, these other food items. A very frequent observation is that cigarette smokers find it much easier to give up smoking on a low-risk food allergy diet than they would on a normal diet. One reason for this may be the absence of cross-reacting to and cross-masking foods from the same family.

Of great interest is the relationship of sugars to the smoking problem. Most physicians working in this field have noted a high incidence of sugar allergy/addiction in cigarette smokers. Some of the addiction to tobacco appears to be related to sugar and to illustrate this one has only to cite the well-known phenomenon in which people who are trying to give up smoking transfer their affections to other forms of sugar such as confectionery.

American blended cigarettes are manufactured from a blend of flue-cured, burley, and oriental tobaccos. Sugars, liquorice, and coca are added in a process which is known as casing. Further 'top-dressing' flavours are usually applied. The precise recipes for casing and flavours are closely guarded by the manufacturers. Therefore, in the case of American blended cigarettes, the allergy/addiction may be predominantly due to the sugars. In these cases the person who ceases smoking but continues with a diet still containing sugar keeps the sugar addiction going, but is deliberately avoiding the twenty or more masking effects that cigarette smoking normally affords. Also, as cigarette smoke is inhaled, the masking occurs very much more rapidly than when sugar is ingested. In these circumstances, it is no wonder that cigarette smokers find it hard to give up smoking. If, however, they go on to a hypo-allergenic diet at the same time, they will of course avoid concurrently inhaled and ingested sugar and in my experience by about day 5 on such a diet, most patients find that their addiction to cigarettes has pretty well ceased.

In the case of cigarettes originating in the UK, the situation is rather different. The cigarettes are usually manufactured from flue-cured tobacco without any additives. The flue-cured tobacco typically contains approximately 15–20 per cent natural sugar. This sugar is a dextrose-type sugar, but unlike the dextrose in our diet, it is not manufactured from corn and therefore it is unlikely (as far as we know at present) to cross-react with other sugars in our diet.

In the case of cigars originating in the UK there are no additives, but many cigars from other sources, for example the USA, have added materials such as sugar.

Pipe tobacco in the UK is made from both flue-cured and burley tobaccos. Sugars are usually added in the form of glucose, fructose, or sucrose. Rum and other flavouring materials are also frequently added. In the USA the additives are similar.

Therefore, to summarize the relationship between smoking and arthritis, I can say: (1) I have never seen an arthritic patient clear all problems by giving up smoking alone; (2) cigarettes, cigars and pipe tobacco may all contain items which can cross-react with and cross-mask other items in the diet, and so these items need to be avoided concurrently with the avoidance of the tobacco; (3) while on a strict diet such as above and avoiding cigarettes, the resumption of cigarette smoking has frequently been observed to cause the re-appearance of arthritic symptoms; (4) for all these reasons it is usually much easier to stop cigarette smoking on a low-risk food allergy diet than it is while on a normal diet containing items such as potatoes, tomatoes, peppers, and the various sugars.

5 Inhaled allergies and arthritis

For many years it has been known that asthma and perennial rhinitis (constant runny or blocked nose) are frequently caused by inhaled air-borne allergens, such as house dust, dust-mites, animal furs, atmospheric moulds, feathers, and so on. Hay fever is of course always caused by air-borne summer pollens.

Only recently, however, have some physicians discovered that arthritis can be partly influenced by such air-borne factors. On taking histories from patients with arthritis one frequently hears:

- My arthritis is enormously improved if I take a holiday in a hot dry climate such as in the Mediterranean area.
- My arthritis is much worse when the weather is damp.
- My arthritis is decidedly worse just before a thunderstorm. I can even tell from my joints when it is about to rain.

In hot dry climates, especially semi-desert areas like the Costa del Sol in Spain and the more arid Greek Islands, there is a very low incidence of inhaled allergy problems. To start with, most of the accommodation has tiled or marbled floors without carpets. Carpets are far and away the biggest source of house dust and house dust mite. The high temperatures found in these areas also discourage dust mite, even in the bedding mattresses. Atmospheric moulds also do not thrive well in hot dry climates and much prefer cool damp conditions such as are found in the United Kingdom. In damp weather, particularly in the summer, the mould count in the atmosphere increases, and it increases spectacularly just before a thunderstorm. There is good reason to believe that this rise in the mould count is the cause of the increased pain that some arthritic sufferers experience just before a thunderstorm. Of course, before thunderstorms other things change, such as barometric pressure and ionization, but it is thought that the mould count, which can increase over 20-fold in the few hours before a thunderstorm, is the most important factor. The evidence we have for this is that individuals do not seem to experience this problems after taking neutralization therapy to specific moulds.

Other potential inhaled allergens may also be left at home when one patient travels to a hot dry climate. Obviously, cats and dogs are usually left when travelling abroad because of quarantine and other problems. One may also be leaving one's feather pillow or wool carpets, both of which can cause potential problems. It must also be remembered that one may also be avoiding chemical problems when one travels to the Mediterranean, such as gas or formaldehyde, which have been dealt with in detail in Chapter 4.

The good news is that neutralization therapy, using extracts of inhaled allergens, usually produced the same remarkable beneficial results that we see when we are dealing with food sensitivities (see Chapter 10). As with food neutralization, the benefit occurs within a matter of a week or so and sometimes even within a couple of days.

Clearly, if a patient with arthritis has an inhaled allergy, neutralization is almost always essential as there is often no way of avoiding these air-borne problems. Certainly the contact with house dust and dust mite can be enormously reduced by changing one's house to look like a Mediterranean villa. Carpets would need to be replaced by tiles or linoleum. Bedding mattresses should be enclosed in polythene bags. Soft furnishings are kept to a minimum. Curtains should be washable and washed frequently.

These changes can markedly reduce the problem at home, but what about the problem at work, for example? The mould count can be reduced in the house using mould retardants to reduce the moulds around windows, under the sink, and so forth, but there is a mould count in the outdoor air which it is impossible to influence. Therefore, for most people neutralization therapy is the only practical solution short of emigrating to a hot dry climate.

Case histories

For some people the inhaled allergy problem seems to be the main one, and a good example of this was Kelvin S. This man was 36 when he first attended my clinic. He had been referred by his consultant rheumatologist to investigate the possibility that his rheumatoid arthritis (seropositive) could be at least partially related to allergy. The condition had been present for five years and was becoming progressively worse and, as he told me later, he was beginning to think in terms of buying himself a wheelchair.

When he first attended he was taking 30mg of Prednisolone (cortisone) each day. Both feet, knees, hips, shoulders, and his right elbow were painful, swollen, and stiff. The history was quite suggestive of food sensitivity and what made it even more likely was the observation that if he ate orange and lemon his joints, which were painful anyway, became even more so. On the usual elimination diet there was a distinct but partial improvement in his symptoms, but he reported that there was still a lot of residual pain, particularly bad first thing in the morning but becoming almost non-existent by early evening.

This pattern of symptoms is usually suggestive of reactions to house dust and house dust mite. Contact with dust and dust mite is high in most bedrooms and therefore patients who react to these items are at their worst first thing in the morning after spending the whole night in this environment. As they go about their business during the day, the contact is usually much less and symptoms begin to wane. Accordingly we tested Kelvin for these allergies using the intradermal provocative technique. Both house dust and dust mite showed strong skin reactions and we went on to determine the specific neutralizing doses.

The first injection of his neutralizing levels of dust and dust mite had the most enormous effect on him. The following morning this man who was on the verge of buying himself a wheelchair went out and played football with his children, something he had not done for several years. Within 24 hours he had changed from about 40 per cent improved to over 90 per cent improved. In the next few weeks he sorted out his specific food reactions which were to wheat, corn, oats, rye, malt, soy, Cheddar cheese, lamb and beef. Meanwhile we were continuing steadily to reduce his cortisone and after a few more weeks he was able to stop it altogether. He has never taken it since.

What was remarkable about this patient was the large role that dust and dust mite allergy played in his problems. He took neutralizing injections for these items for a few months and then found that he no longer needed them unless he got into situations of very high dust and dust mite contamination.

Two years after his initial work-out, he told me that he had remained very well since. As he personally did not like taking the minute injections he had decided to avoid the foods to which he was sensitive but he had already developed a partial tolerance to them. He was finding that as long as he ate his food allergens only about one day in four he no longer reacted. If he ate them more frequently than this he would do.

In a letter to his consultant a few months after starting his treatment with us he wrote,

> *Thank you very much for referring me because the results are unbelievable and it is a terrible shame that this treatment is not available to those who need it because of the restrictions imposed by the National Health Service.*

Many people, after sorting out their food sensitivities, find that their main joint pain and swelling have abated but their morning stiffness and discomfort may still remain to some extent. The main contact with house dust and house dust mite occurs while we lie in our beds asleep at night, on a mattress usually thick with house dust mites. Dust mites are so small that they cannot even be seen with an ordinary microscrope and it is their faeces which cause the allergic reaction. Most bedrooms are also heavily carpeted. Any symptom, therefore, associated with dust and dust mite exposure tends to be at its worst on awakening in the morning.

It was Dr Michael Radcliffe, one of the founder members of the British Society for Allergy and Environmental Medicine, who first alerted me to the possibility that inhaled allergens such as house dust could be so important in arthritis. He told me of several of his patients who had residual morning stiffness and pain despite eliminating their food sensitivities. On skin testing he had found some of them to be sensitive to house dust and dust mite and after neutralization therapy these remaining symptoms had disappeared. I tested several of my patients with the same residual symptoms and many of them responded in the same way.

A case in which dust and dust mite allergy played a minor but important role was Mary M. This patient, aged 49, first attended my clinic in 1986 with her husband, Carlos. They had three grown-up children, and Mary and Carlos had been happily planning their future together in a little house in a mountain village in Carlos's native Italy. Unhappily in 1983 the future started to look bleak as Mary began to develop joint pain after joint pain, and her husband became worried that the once lovely wife that he had would be a crippled old lady by the time they got to their retirement home in Italy.

Initially Mary had a painful, swollen hand and her GP referred her to the local hospital, where she was found to have a high sedimentation rate which is suggestive of rheumatoid arthritis. She was prescribed Naproxen and this gave some relief initially. Three months later her other hand began to show similar symptoms and the Naproxen was no longer giving the relief it did at first. Cortisone injections were given into the worst affected joints which provided some help. About this time Mary was also requested by the hospital to take part in a clinical trial, in respect of a new arthritis drug from America. This drug did not help her at all and she was not even told the final results of the trial.

Her full-time job as a chef in a private school in London was now becoming too much for Mary to hold down. Her feet had become affected and were swollen and painful most of the time. She was fatigued after very little exertion and her husband was relieved when Mary decided that the full-time job was a thing of the past for her. In addition to the symptoms already mentioned, Mary had quite a lot of rhinitis (continuous runny nose) and some headaches and migraines. At about this time Mary read that anti-inflammatory drugs such as Naproxen were getting a lot of bad press, and not without reason as they had been found to be causing severe side-effects in many people. As they were not really giving her any relief now from pain and swelling she decided to stop taking them.

About this time she heard from a neighbour who had arthritis about allergy testing, and as this neighbour had received considerable benefit she made an appointment to see me at the clinic. As she said later, the day she attended the clinic was a turning point in her life. When I took her history she told me that the one time that her rheumatoid arthritis had been really good was when she went to Italy on a vist to her husband's home town. She felt so good in Italy, in fact, that she had not needed to take drugs while she was there. This, combined with the fact that she had a rhinitis problem, alerted me very much to the possibility that reactions to house dust and house dust mite were important in her case.

Accordingly we started off by testing her for these items and as expected she was strongly positive. We gave her the injections for a few days before we put her on the elimination diet and within those few days her runny nose problem virtually disappeared. There was also some improvement in her joints. On the second, third and fourth day of the elimination diet she had a very classic withdrawal response. She felt so ill on these days that she stayed in bed. By the sixth day she went into work to be told by everyone how well she looked. She told her workmates that her fingers could move, she could lift her arms above her head and she could get her shoes on to her feet without discomfort. When I saw her on the seventh day I told her to reintroduce foods back into her diet. She had strong reactions to beef and milk and milder reactions to wheat, corn and lemon. She knew, incidentally, before she attended the clinic that orange and grapefruit tended to make her worse than usual.

In the two years since initially attending the clinic she has remained extremely well. She has continued in full-time employment and she only has the most minimal occasional symptoms in her joints. She is able to do aerobics and her earlier problems are now just one nasty memory. She took her neutralizing injections for dust and dust mite for some time and has now discontinued them. She is, however, still aware that heavy exposure to old, dusty places can still bring on some joint pain. She has sensibly changed her bedding and furnishings to items that attract the minimum of house dust and dust mite.

Unlike the previous case history, I estimate that only about 30 per cent of Mary's arthritis symptoms were related to the inhalation of house dust and dust mite, but this is more typical of the patients that we see. However, to improve someone with rheumatoid arthritis from 70 per cent to almost 100 per cent as a result of about two hours of skin testing and a few neutralizing injections is, I think, a very worthwhile use of medical resources.

To conclude, it seems that all inhaled allergens can be implicated in the cause of arthritis.

In one remarkable patient we obtained an approximate 50 per cent general improvement in her condition by sorting out her food sensitivities. This, by her own estimate, improved to 75 per cent by neutralization therapy for house dust and dust mites. Most of the other inhalants we tested were negative. However, cat dander was decidedly positive and when we arrived at her neutralizing concentration of cat dander she was able to completely close her fist for the first time for several years. She owned four cats, and adding the cat neutralization to her injection treatment produced almost total improvement. She did not even have to say goodbye to the cats.

6 Intestinal candidiasis

Some individuals may go on to a low-risk allergy diet and not improve at all. They may also be tested for inhaled allergens like house dust, house dust mite, and moulds with negative results. They may be tested for chemical sensitivity, again with negative results. They might even go into an environmental control unit and fast for five days, and still show no improvement in their arthritis. This is rare, but it does occur and at one time these patients were regarded as failures of this form of arthritis management.

Obviously the cause of these people's arthritis lies outside the normal realm of reactions to foods, chemicals, or inhalants. My first clue to this missing cause was a lecture by Dr Orion Truss at the 15th Advanced Seminar of the Society for Clinical Ecology, in Atlanta, Georgia, concerning the relationship of thrush to human illness. Thrush is an organism that most people have heard about: its proper medical name is *Candida albicans*. Up to the time of this meeting I had throught of this organism as causing only vaginal thrush in adult females and oral thrush most frequently in the mouths of babies. Both conditions are usually easily cured by short courses of anti-fungicides and, except in a few unfortunate adult females where the condition could recur with monotonous frequency, it was not thought of as a major problem. Also, like all doctors, I knew that the whole of the intestinal tract was normally colonized by Candida organisms but they appeared to cause no problem. This is still, I should emphasize, the view held by most of the medical profession.

What Dr Orion Truss said was that this view was wrong and that intestinal thrush could cause a huge array of medical problems, varying quite considerably in symptom pattern from one person to another. He also said that the problem was extremely common and was a major cause of human illness. Dr Truss is, I might add, a physician of considerable standing and has served as Instructor in Medicine at Cornell Medical College and Instructor in Clinical Medicine at the University of Alabama Medical College, amongst other major appointments.

What this physician had in fact discovered was another basic cause of illness. Not only could people respond adversely to the foods, chemicals, and inhalants that they encountered, but they could also react to the microflora of their intestinal tract. Although it did not occur to me at the time, it was an obvious possible explanation of why patients with chronic illness that appeared to be environmentally induced might not improve in an environmental control unit. The patient may say goodbye to foods, chemicals, and inhalants on entering such a unit, but the gut and its flora are still there.

Having spent many years researching the role of candidiasis in human illness, Dr Truss reported his observations in three separate papers in the *Journal of Orthomolecular Medicine*. These papers did not make a great impact on the medical profession in general, mostly I think because physicians could not perceive how these findings could fit in with their other knowledge and medical practice. However, physicians in the allergy field who were looking at illness purely in terms of cause and effect, as opposed to naming a disease and attempting to suppress it, knew they had been missing a major cause of illness and so this work fell on much more receptive ears in their case.

At this point I must emphasize that in my experience direct problems with intestinal candidiasis play an important but comparatively small role in arthritis and this view is shared by other doctors working in the field. If I were to write a book on irritable bowel syndrome, Crohn's disease, migraine, urticaria, or eczema, for example, I would devote maybe a third of the book to this problem and in the case of psoriasis I would devote the whole book to it (see Chapter 7).

The Candida phenomenon

Like most of life, the whole Candida problem centres around balance. On one side of the equation is Candida albicans and on the other side is the resistance of the host. Although Candida has in the past been regarded as an innocent commensal of the digestive tract, mycology (the study of moulds and fungi) has demonstrated that Candida albicans is very complex. It releases at least 79 known chemical substances, against which the human body creates an identifiable antibody. There are in fact 81 strains of Candida albicans and each strain can produce 35 separate antigens. Varying strains can colonize the gut of the same person at different times in his or her life. A healthy individual has these organisms present only in small quantities in the gastro-intestinal tract and in such people no harm results.

Candida albicans is an opportunistic organism. It will grow spectacularly when an individual's resistance is lowered or when it is particularly encouraged by factors occurring in someone's lifestyle. Resistance can be lowered by an infection, nutritional deficiencies, or some debilitating agent in the environment. Factors in our modern lifestyle that are important are high consumption of antibiotics, the contraceptive pill, and cortisone. High sugar and yeast consumption are very important, especially the sugar consumption.

When conditions are ripe for Candida proliferation it tends to change in shape from its normal yeast-like form to a mycelial fungal form. Candida albicans is thus called a dimorphic organism because it can exist in two separate shapes. The yeast-like form is thought to be non-invasive and probably harmless. The fungal form, however, has long root-like mycelia which can penetrate the mucous membrane lining of the intestines. This penetration of the mucosal lining can lead to 'leaky' mucous membranes and this can be seen with an electron microscope. Such a leaky mucosa is of enormous importance as it can allow incompletely digested dietary proteins, etc. to come into direct contact with the immune system. The outposts of the immune system lie underneath the mucosa and they are designed to deal with food that has been broken down by digestive enzymes and is thus of low molecular weight. The contact between the immune system and these unbroken-down foodstuffs is an obvious mechanism for the production of food allergy or sensitivity. Hence patients who have a chronic overgrowth of Candida albicans and a high percentage of the mycelial form frequently show a wide variety of food and environmental allergies.

Patients with multiple food and chemical sensitivities may become that way because antibodies were formed to the antigenic proteins in foods, pollens and even, importantly, to their own intestinal flora. In addition to causing a leaky mucosa it has now been convincingly demonstrated (see Chapter 14) that Candida produces a specific toxin called Candida toxin which seems to weaken the immune system in general and make it less able to cope with other allergy problems. In particular, Candida toxin suppresses the T-lymphocytes in our immune defence systems and, as these cells are the 'generals' of that system, the immune system tends to perform in a rather disorganized manner. It is thought that when neutralization therapy for food and inhalant allergies (see Chapter 11) is not working well, it is usually due to a poorly functioning immune system and is accompanied by depressed levels of T-lymphocytes. Many failures of neutralization become successes after Candida treatment.

Candida treatment is thought to lead to a reduction in gut permeability and it is very noticcable clinically that further food sensitivities seem much less likely to occur. In difficult, complex, refractory-type patients, Candida treatment tends to stabilize them and make them easier to treat. Minor food sensitivities often disappear and neutralization levels (see Chapter 11) remain much more stable.

Diagnosis

The diagnosis that chronic intestinal candidiasis is important in a specific patient is based on the whole clinical picture, established by taking a history from the patient. There are currently in the USA various experimental blood tests described in detail in the book *The Yeast Syndrome* by Dr J.P. Trowbridge and Morton Walker (Bantam Books). They include a Candida Antigen Profile, the Candi-sphere Serodiagnostic Analysis, and the Candida albicans Antibody Titer Test. These tests are undergoing long-term evaluation at the moment and may be found to be very helpful when this evaluation is complete.

In arthritis sufferers, the starting point for the diagnosis is often the absence of beneficial response to food, chemical and inhalant management. In such people, it is thought that the arthritic symptoms are caused as a direct result of the production of Candida toxin. If the Candida problem were just predisposing the patient to food sensitivity, then an elimination diet would have produced at least some benefit.

If, in addition, symptoms such as those following are observed, I would be further encouraged in my diagnosis and would embark on a course of aggressive treatment for candidiasis. If the patient responds to this treatment, the diagnosis is confirmed. Thus a therapeutic trial, which is well known and respected in other areas of medicine, is the only ultimate test.

The classic clinical picture consists of the existence of: (a) predisposing factors; and (b) clinical symptoms.

Factors which predispose to chronic intestinal candidiasis are: (1) Recurrent or prolonged treatment with antibiotics. All physicians know that antibiotics stir up intestinal candidiasis, but what they are not so universally aware of is the long-term adverse effects that can thereby accrue. The worst antibiotics in this respect are the broad-spectrum antibiotics such as tetracycline. These antibiotics kill a lot of the more innocent microorganisms in the digestive tract and thereby encourage Candida albicans. The worst single example of this is the current frequent practice of treating teenage acne with courses of tetracycline, often extending over several years. I have seen many patients who have had severe problems after such treatment.

(2) Prolonged use of the contraceptive pill. The pill is an immunosuppressive drug and, as Dr Ellen Grant frequently points out, is a steroid — in other words a cortisone-like drug. As a result Dr Grant, who has spent much of her medical career researching the contraceptive pill, insists on calling oral contraceptives the 'oral contraceptive steroid' to emphasize this point. I think she is right because both doctors and patients frequently lose sight of the fact that the patients are actually taking a steroid. Steroids work basically by suppressing the immune system and anything that suppresses the immune system will allow Candida to proliferate more easily.

(3) Prolonged treatment with Cortisone or cortisone-derived drugs for any particular reason.

(4) Multiple pregnancies.

(5) An environment containing a high proportion of mould. There is a fascinating interaction between environmental moulds and Candida albicans. People with severe candidiasis frequently are particularly bad in the mould season of the year, which in the UK is August, September, and early October. These individuals tend to be particularly bad on damp, humid days in August and September when the mould count is clearly high. They will frequently be improved dramatically by desensitization to moulds in addition to their Candida treatment. If a sufferer lives in a damp house with a lot of mould on the walls in the bathroom and in the kitchen, steps should be taken to eradicate these moulds as far as possible. Various techniques have been described in relation to this, but they are beyond the

scope of this book.

(6) A history of high consumption of sugar in the past. A lot of Candida sufferers crave sugar in any form and in fact it is one of the diagnostic features of the condition. Frequently the craving amounts to a total addiction.

(7) Ingestion of large quantities of yeast products.

It will be noticed that all these predisposing factors, with the exception of environmental moulds and pregnancies, are items which have steadily increased with advancing civilization.

Yeast started to be used by human beings about 8,000 years ago, but only in a small way. Nowadays yeast products occur prolifically in our diet. Yeast is present in all leavened breads, all alcoholic beverages, most cheeses, mushrooms, and most fruit juices. The consumption of sugar, which was totally unknown in Europe prior to the sixteenth century, has increased spectacularly throughout this century and the consumption of sugar per head of the population has increased over thirty-fold since the beginning of the twentieth century.

Antibiotics have been with us to some extent since 1942, but most of the broad-spectrum antibiotics did not arrive until the mid and late 1940s. Cortisone and the contraceptive pill began to be used in the 1950s. All these items are now being used in progressively increasing quantities.

Symptoms suggestive of intestinal candidiasis

Candida can lead to an enormous range of symptom manifestations. The commonest and most characteristic symptoms are:

- bloating and gaseous distention of the abdomen
- chronic rectal irritation
- repeated or chronic thrush vaginitis
- recurrent bouts of what is frequently called cystitis, when it is in fact cystourethritis (bacteriological cultures of the urine are negative and there is no direct specific evidence of Candida albicans because the infection is deep in the cells of the urethra and bladder)
- recurring depression, irritability, inability to concentrate, and problems with memory
- chronic nervous indigestion-symptoms, especially in the upper part of the digestive tract (these symptoms are often erroneously diagnosed as hiatus hernia)

- chronic constipation, sometimes alternating with diarrhoea
- recurring fungal-type rashes in different parts of the body.
  Virtually nobody has all these symptoms and of course they can be the result of processes other than Candida. The presence of a fair number of these symptoms is highly suggestive of the problem, but what absolutely clinches the diagnosis is that these symptoms are aggravated by factors which classically aggravate thrush — in other words, they are often made worse by courses of antibiotics or high consumption of sugar and yeast.

Treatment

The treatment of chronic intestinal candidiasis is usually a fairly prolonged business and at times can be quite difficult. Practitioners currently use one of the following five methods: (1) Nystatin plus diet; (2) caprylic acid plus diet; (3) Nizoral plus diet; (4) Amphotericin-B plus diet; and (5) Lactobacillus acidophilus plus diet. Diet is extremely important in the treatment of candidiasis, probably about half the total treatment. Intestinal thrush is quite resistant to treatment and so we have to starve the thrush out by depriving it of what it thrives on, and attack it with various medications. The absolutely ideal diet to combat thrush would contain no carbohydrates at all, but this would be dangerous to the general health of the individual. The diet therefore represents a reasonable compromise between the nutritional needs of the individual and the speed with which the ultimate result needs to be attained. The degree of restriction also of course depends to some extent on the severity of the individual's Candida problem.

All physicians who have treated this problem are agreed that sugar is the most important item to be avoided. This food is the most easily available source of nutrition for Candida, which proliferates rapidly when it can obtain sugar. All sugars should be restricted and this includes cane sugar, beet sugar, glucose, powdered fructose, honey, and maple syrup. I allow my patients to eat some fruits which of course contain fructose, but I instruct them to eat only those that contain the least fructose.

Having experimented with varying degrees of restriction, I have now settled on the following initial diet, which although fairly restrictive, usually leads to obvious improvement if combined with an effective anti-fungal medication in about two to three months. If the diet is less restrictive, improvement usually takes longer, and if that happens one might run into a 'credibility gap'.

Therefore, for most people I recommend the following diet for approximately two months, although they may let up on it a bit if obvious improvement occurs within a few weeks.

Anti-Candida Diet
Phase 1

To be followed for 8 weeks

The following foods *only* to be eaten:

cabbage
cauliflower
broccoli
spring greens
spinach
curly kale
carrots
parsnips
swede
courgettes (zucchini)
marrow
red and green peppers
aubergine (eggplant)
leek
onion
garlic
shallots
celery
celeriac
pumpkin
bamboo shoots
bean sprouts
water chestnuts
ginger
chicory
kohl rabi
okra
mung bean sprouts
salsify
parsley
chives
globe artichoke
Jerusalem artichoke
Brussels sprouts

peas — not petits pois
mangetout
kelp (seaweed)
runner beans
French beans
asparagus
lettuce
cucumber
radish
tomato
Chinese leaves
watercress
all fresh or dried herbs, eg.
thyme, sage, oregano, clove,
cumin, turmeric, rosemary,
nutmeg, etc.
Tabasco sauce
potatoes
potato flour
rice
rice cakes
rice flour
cornflour (corn starch)

sunflower oil
sunflower seed
tahini
sesame oil
sesame seed
olives
cold-pressed olive oil
cold-pressed linseed oil
safflower oil
butter (in moderation)

beef including all offal
lamb including all offal
pork including all offal
rabbit
chicken including eggs
turkey
duck including eggs
veal
venison
pheasant and all game birds

shellfish including:
crab
lobster
prawns
shrimps
oysters
cockles
winkles
mussels
scallops
whelks

All saltwater and freshwater fish
(*not* breaded) including:
cod
plaice
trout
haddock
sole
hake
salmon
eel
halibut
monkfish
sea bass
tuna
turbot
sardines

herrings
mackerel

split peas
black-eyed peas
chick-peas
chick-pea flour

avocado
rhubarb
lemon
lime
guava
melon

goats' milk
goats' yoghurt
live cows' milk yoghurt
Edam cheese
Gouda cheese
soft cream cheese
cottage cheese

soya beans
soya milk
soya flour
soya oil
tofu

Drink only the following:

jasmine tea
green tea
herbal teas
carrot juice (bottled or fresh)
tomato juice (bottled or fresh)
goats' milk
soya milk
water

Once there has been some improvement, which should usually
occur in about eight to twelve weeks, you can then expand your
dietary repertoire into the Phase 2 Anti-Candida Diet.

Phase 2

To be followed for 10 weeks

The following foods to be added to those on Phase 1:

wheat (soda bread can be made using wholemeal flour and bicarbonate of soda)
oats
barley
rye
buckwheat
sweetcorn
fresh ground coffee
full cream cows' milk
lentils
dried peas

dried beans and all pulses from health food shops
satsuma, strawberry
apple, cherry, blackberry
gooseberry, peach, pineapple, pomegranate

almond
chestnut
filbert   To be eaten only in small quantities
hazelnut
peanut

In most individuals, improvement continues on this diet and in a further two to three months they can expand into Phase 3, which returns the diet to almost normal, with the notable exception of the sugar products.

Phase 3

To be followed for 10 weeks

It may now be possible for you to introduce some yeast-related foods into your diet.

To test your sensitivity to yeast, take 3 brewer's yeast tablets and note any adverse reactions that may occur over the next two days. If no adverse reaction occurs you may introduce into your diet the following foods:

wholemeal bread
all cheeses
Indian tea   to be eaten in moderation
vinegar
mushrooms

vodka
Scotch whisky   to be taken in moderation with low calorie tonic if wished
gin

You may also introduce:

all other fruits

coconut

Brazil nut
cashew nut
pecan
pistachio
walnut

plus any other foods *not* containing sugar (dextrose/glucose/sucrose/fructose) or honey.

Be very careful to look at all labels on every pre-packaged food product you buy.

As long as you are well, sugar is allowed at times in small quantities, and if you do not wish to see a return of the original problems you are advised to keep your sugar consumption low pretty well for the rest of your life. Low sugar consumption means indulging in a few sauces, curries, and maybe occasional confectionery, but no major return to added sugar in tea or coffee, cakes, biscuits, etc. With the ever-increasing evidence that sugar is involved in a whole host of other major human illnesses, such as coronary artery disease (see Professor John Yudkin's book entitled *Pure White and Deadly*, published by Penguin, 1988) sugar restriction is therefore pretty good advice for anyone interested in their health.

Nystatin

The most effective medication to reduce the colonies of Candida albicans is Nystatin. Nystatin has been used by doctors for over thirty years and has an enviable safety record. This safety record is partly due to the fact that, except at very high dosage, it is not absorbed at all from the alimentary canal. In other words, it does not reach the bloodstream, but remains inside the digestive tract, where it does all its work, killing the yeast germs situated therein. An illustration of the safety of this medication comes from the cancer institutes in America, where some children have been found to be suffering from virulent intestinal candidiasis as a result of the cytotoxic drugs that they have been given. Doses of 100 tablets a day or more of Nystatin have been used to treat these conditions and have been found to be perfectly well tolerated. Nystatin is arguably the safest medication in the British pharmacopoeia.

Most of the doctors I know use pure Nystatin powder rather than Nystatin tablets, which are obtainable at the chemist. I use pure Nystatin powder because: (1) it is much cheaper than the tablets which, when the full dosage is obtained, can be prohibitively expensive; (2) the Candida organisms colonize the whole digestive tract from the mouth to the rectum and, of course, tablets which are swallowed will not treat the organisms in the mouth or the oesophagus; (3) the tablets contain food colourings and other chemicals and filling agents, such as cornflour — these can contribute to the allergy problems or compromise an elimination diet; (4) worst of all, the tablets are sugar-coated, which somewhat defeats a sugar-free diet.

The Nystatin powder must be stored in a refrigerator, but not in the freezer compartment. The most usual regimen is to start taking Nystatin at a dosage of half a level teaspoon per day. The teaspoon should be a 5ml plastic measuring teaspoon. The half-teaspoon dosage is placed into any cold drink that does not contain sugar or yeast and stirred well until it dissolves. This total daily dose of half a teaspoon is taken in four equal doses and spread at roughly equal intervals throughout the day. Ideally the powder should be taken an hour or two before food is ingested. After a week, if there are no problems, the dosage is increased to three-quarters of a teaspoon. In most cases, the dose is thereafter increased by one-quarter of a teaspoon every week until a total dosage of 2½ teaspoons a day is attained.

The Herxheimer response (die-off reaction)

This is the name given to certain problems that can occur with some people as the dose of Nystatin is increased. The problems do not occur only with Nystatin but can occur with any medication that is effectively killing Candida organisms. The more effective the medication, the more likely is the problem to occur.

In some individuals, as the dosage of Nystatin is increased they may, at a certain dosage level, notice a sudden increase in the severity of the very symptoms they are treating. Sometimes, in addition, headache, fatigue, depression, and flu-like symptoms may also make an appearance. The symptoms are almost certainly caused by a sudden large increase in the production of Candida toxin. Nystatin kills Candida germs quite brutally and in laboratory tests it can be shown that the cell wall of Candida albicans disintegrates, releasing the Candida toxin held within that cell wall. Therefore, if large quantities of Candida are killed there is a large release of Candida toxin in the digestive tract.Candida toxin is absorbed from the digestive tract into the bloodstream and can lead to symptoms in any part of the body.

When the dosage of Nystatin is lowered by about half a teaspoon the symptoms will usually die away in three or four days. After another week or two of Nystatin treatment at the slightly reduced dosage the individual will then usually be able to tolerate the dosage of Nystatin which previously produced the Herxheimer response, as more of the Candida germs have now been eliminated.

This response is named after Dr Herxheimer, who in the early part of this century described a similar response when patients were being successfully treated for syphilis. In the cases he observed the syphilitic lesions could be shown to regress but the patient often started to experience joint pains and fever due to the toxin released by the dead spirochaetes (syphilis germs).

Anyone experiencing this type of response can be virtually certain that they have a Candida problem, as people without the Candida problem have no trouble at all in taking any reasonable dose of Nystatin. I have always though that obvious Herxheimer responses are probably the single most certain positive diagnostic indicator of the Candida problem.

There are some people, it must be said, who have a great deal of trouble getting on at all with Nystatin. These are usually those who look pale and ill, with multiple food and chemical sensitivities. They can have decidedly adverse reactions to even microdoses of Nystatin and usually need, at least initially, to be treated with small doses of something like caprylic acid or Lactobacillus acidophilus. There are a few people who will even have Herxheimer reactions to these milder regimes and need to be treated with diet only for a month or two before active treatment can be initiated.

Various manoeuvres can be tried in this type of person to get them through the early stages of effective anti-Candida treatment.

1. Candida neutralization. The technique entails finding a neutralizing level of Candida albicans in the same way as other neutralization therapy (see Chapter 10). The patient then takes daily subcutaneous injections of Candida extract which can produce a considerable immediate symptom improvement and seem to counteract the Herxheimer reaction. In some patients, however, the neutralizing level is rather unstable and has to be adjusted frequently.

2. Temporarily (for about 10–14 days) eliminate all carbohydrate from the diet while rapidly increased doses of Nystatin are taken and in these circumstances the doses can be well-tolerated.

3. Colonic wash-outs to eliminate excess Candida from the colonic area where they are usually at their most prolific.

Ketoconazole

Another chemical approach to this subject is the use of the drug Ketoconazole, which is sold in the UK under the trade name of Nizoral. There are definitely some people who seem to tolerate this drug much better than they do Nystatin. I tend to use the drug only in comparatively short courses, as its safety with prolonged administration has not really been demonstrated. Even using the drug for short courses there is a slight (about 1 in 10,000) risk of hepatitis, and blood tests for liver function need to be performed at regular intervals if this drug is to be used for anything over a few weeks. Ketoconazole, unlike Nystatin, is absorbed from the digestive tract and is carried by the blood circulation to the rest of the body. Consequently it will treat Candida germs in the skin, vagina, and any other tissues. I have a general impression that it seems to kill Candida a little less dramatically and more smoothly than Nystatin and that patients taking it are often less likely to have a Herxheimer reaction. To summarize, therefore, Nizoral is a useful second-string medication for this problem. Personally I have never had any major problem prescribing it, but it does not have as exceptional a safety record as Nystatin.

Amphotericin-B

This is an anti-fungal antibiotic which has a mode of action identical to that of Nystatin. Like Nystatin, it is not absorbed from the gut except in extremely high dosage. Data from many sources indicate that this drug is a safe alternative to Nystatin and can be valuable: (a) to those who do not tolerate Nystatin; (b) to those having a poor clinical response to Nystatin; or (c) to those who symptomatically relapse while taking Nystatin, despite an initial apparent improvement.

Amphotericin-B is currently available in the UK and is retailed under the trade name of Fungilin in 100mg tablets. I usually try to work up to the maximum dosage suggested by the makers, which is 2 100mg tablets four times a day.

In hospital practice Amphotericin-B is sometimes given by intravenous injection. Giving it this way is very effective in treating Candida in deeper tissues but is, however, decidedly dangerous leading to possible kidney damage. I would only advocate the tablet form of the medication which is almost totally safe.

Caprylic acid

This anti-fungal medication is a short-chain fatty acid originally discovered over thirty years ago by Dr Irene Neuhauser of the University of Illinois. The huge recent upsurge in interest in candidiasis prompted various companies to dig up old research on anti-fungal substances and this particular item has proved to be very useful. Caprylic acid is now retailed by different companies as Capricin Forte, Caprystatin, and Kapricidin-A, etc. My current favourite is Capricin Forte which seems to work exceptionally well in many people, possibly because it becomes uniformally dispersed on the gut wall along the entire length of the intestine. The therapeutic dosage is 9 capsules of Capricin Forte daily, 3 capsules taken three times a day with meals to maximize the fungal effect and minimize the belching which sometimes occurs.

As caprylic acid is extremely safe, it is retailed as a food supplement. Hence it can be bought over the counter at health food shops and is often advocated by naturopaths, chiropractors, etc. unlike Nystatin, Nizoral, or Amphotericin-B, which are of course available only on a doctor's prescription. The manufacturers of Capricin suggest that its value may be enhanced if a high-yield Lactobacillus acidophilus preparation is given at the same time. As with any other product that kills Candida effectively, it can of course lead to the Herxheimer or die-off reaction, and as with the other medications, the problem can usually be solved by temporarily reducing the dosage and then gradually increasing it again after more of the Candida cells have been eradicated. It is noticeable that the Herxheimer reactions with this product tend to be milder and less frequent.

Lactobacillus acidophilus

A non-chemical approach to Candida is the use of Lactobacillus acidophilus. This is a micro-organism which normally resides in the digestive tract of all people. On average an adult will have approximately 2½lb of various micro-organisms present in the lower small intestine and colon. Lactobacillus acidophilus figures prominently in this population of micro-organisms and is wholly beneficial. There are over 200 known strains of Lactobacillus acidophilus. Only one strain has marked anti-Candida activity and this has been marketed in the UK in products such as Superdophilus and Primodophilus. Superdophilus has a guaranteed one billion live Lactobacillus acidophilus germs per gram and is a much more potent and effective product than some similar products, especially those retailed in tablet form. Lactobacillus acidophilus should be kept refrigerated and never exposed to temperatures above 80°F (26.7°C).

Lactobacillus acidophilus exerts its beneficial influence by actively competing for space on the mucous membranes of the digestive tract with colonies of Candida albicans. It is also thought to have a specific antagonistic effect on the Candida albicans. In general I find Lactobacillus acidophilus works far slower and less dramatically than Nystatin or Nizoral. Its main use, therefore, is in instances when the more potent drugs cannot be tolerated. It also aids beneficial recolonization of the gut after Candida has been largely eliminated.

Oleic acid and biotin

Another couple of products which are non-chemical and helpful in combating candidiasis are oleic acid and biotin. Oleic acid is found in cold-pressed olive oil and linseed oil. It acts by inhibiting the fungal form of Candida albicans and encouraging the yeast form. It is normally taken, for example, as cold-pressed olive oil in a dosage of 2 teaspoons three times a day.

It has been discovered that the conversion from the yeast form of Candida albicans to the mycelial form is partly dependent upon a deficiency of biotin. It is thought that biotin, when given orally, can prevent the conversion of Candida to its mycelial form. It is usually taken in a dosage of 500mcg twice daily.

Garlic

This foodstuff has been used for medicinal purposes for centuries. Many scientific papers have now been published on the effects observed in the laboratory of garlic on strains of Candida albicans. One study, for example, showed that 24 out of 26 strains of Candida albicans were sensitive to aqueous dilutions of garlic extract. No large-scale controlled clinical trials of garlic have ever been conducted or are likely to be. The cost of such trials is huge and if they strongly support the efficacy of garlic as an anti-fungal agent, who is going to make any substantial money out of retailing a substance that cannot be patented? This is a dreadful but mostly true comment on factors that influence medical progress.

Eminent physicians who have studied garlic state that it is a highly effective anti-fungal agent. Amounts small enough on your breath not to create a social problem will have beneficial effects. The major chemical constituent of whole garlic which gives it its therapeutic effectiveness is allicin, which is also unfortunately responsible for the odour of garlic. Removing the allicin to remove the odour will also remove the anti-fungal effect. Garlic powder and whole garlic cloves are undoubtedly effective, but there is a distinct question-mark in my mind as to the effectiveness of the odourless preparations.

There is currently a great deal of discussion as to the various merits and demerits of the anti-fungal substances I have just described. In general, treatment of Candida has fallen into two distinct camps. On one side are the allopathic physicians who are legally entitled to prescribe anti-fungal medications, such as Nystatin, Amphotericin-B and Ketoconazole. These physicians also employ diets similar to the ones I have described earlier in this chapter. Another route is followed by alternative health therapists, such as chiropractors and naturopaths, who are legally unable to prescribe these drugs. They rely on caprylic acid, Lactobacillus acidophilus, garlic, oleic acid and biotin. I, in common with other allopathic physicians, do, however, make quite a lot of use of the more natural anti-fungal medications in patients who are particularly sensitive to the Herxheimer-type response.

Neutralization therapy for candidiasis

Another treatment used by many allergists treating this problem is vaccination using extracts of Candida albicans. I use Candida albicans extract in varying strengths in the same way as I use food or inhalant extracts to neutralize patients to foods or inhalants as described in Chapters 10 and 11. Neutralizing doses of Candida albicans can be spectacularly effective in helping the patient, especially in the short term. The response is sometimes so dramatic that it totally convinces the patient that the problems are related to Candida albicans.

The disadvantage of this treatment is that the neutralizing level of Candida albicans has an awkward habit of changing rather rapidly, necessitating retesting at frequent intervals. Sometimes desensitization with TCE, which is a mixture of trichophyton, Candida albicans, and epidermophyton, can be even more successful. Trichophyton and epidermophyton are two other fungal micro-organisms found in the digestive tract and they cause problems in very much the same way as Candida albicans.

Case histories

I will now discuss three patients whose arthritis has been markedly helped by anti-candidiasis treatment. A major factor suggesting candidiasis in an arthritis sufferer is a negative response to an elimination diet combined with negative skin tests for inhalant sensitivity. If there are also positive signs of candidiasis, the suspicion is further heightened.

Such a patient was Ralph E. who was 51 when he first consulted me. He had a history of joint pain extending back for about 1½ years. The problem started in his right knee and then spread to the rest of the joints in his right leg. The next joints to become involved were his left wrist and elbow, and right thumb which became extremely swollen. He was seen by a rheumatologist and as his serum was negative for rheumatoid factor he was diagnosed as suffering from non-specific polyarthritis.

His GP in Central London, who had for many years taken an active interest in the 'allergy' side of arthritis, tried him on a 'lamb and pear' exclusion diet. After seven days on this diet he showed absolutely no response, either in terms of withdrawal symptoms in the first few days or improvement towards the end of the diet.

When I saw him at my clinic he had very little in his history to indicate food sensitivity, but he had many symptoms suggestive of intestinal candidiasis. The patient had, as he confessed to me, a very sweet tooth with a moderately high sugar consumption. He suffered from considerable wind, bloating, and other indigestion symptoms for which he regularly took Bisodol. There was a distinct long-term history of constipation. Every summer he would suffer from athlete's foot (*tinea pedis*), a classic symptom of fungal overload. His memory, he told me, had deteriorated considerably in the past year or so. However, what really clinched the diagnosis in my mind was a marked and long-standing history of pruritus ani (itching around the anus). Long-standing pruritus ani, I am now convinced (except in the presence of piles), is nearly always a strong indicator of intestinal thrush. Further additions to his diagnostic picture were his observation that petrol fumes would give him a headache and that his joints were improved in Eilat. Hot dry atmospheres have a very low mould count and, although he was later shown not to be allergic to moulds, it is thought that moulds can interreact and stimulate intestinal thrush without the patient being sensitive to them.

As a precaution we first placed him on our Stage I diet (see Chapter 9) just in case he was sensitive to lamb, which we no longer use as a safe food in patients with arthritis. Again, however, he had negative result on this diet and skin tests for house dust, dust-mite, moulds and gas were all negative.

We then placed him on our Phase 1 Candida treatment diet and gave him increasing doses of Nystatin. By the time he had reached the 2½ teaspoon level of Nystatin he was at least 80 per cent better as long as he did not divert from the diet. The pain, swelling and stiffness in the joints of his left hand and elbow had disappeared entirely. The right thumb was only a fraction of the initial problem. His hips showed only slight niggles, which were always associated with distinct diversions from his diet. He was a very decided sugar addict and his diversions were nearly always chocolate.

Now he swims twice a day and follows other very energetic pursuits which he would not even have been able to contemplate a few months previously. His pruritus ani, athlete's foot, weight and memory problems are now also things of the past. I emphasize he was on no other medication than Nystatin.

Another patient sent to me by the same physician was Nigel B., who was 47 when he first attended the clinic. This man's problem was osteoarthritis in his left hip, which had become progressively worse over the preceding seven years and would keep him awake at night. Most nights he would wake up at least five times to try to find a more comfortable position in which to lie. What was particularly interesting in this patient was that he also suffered from psoriasis, which was present predominantly on the back of his scalp, elbows, knees, etc.

Psoriasis is a very nasty skin disorder characterized by large scaling plaques and in patients who have it badly it is one of the most disfiguring skin conditions of all. Until recently nobody had any idea as to what caused the condition, but it has now been linked with candidiasis and we have seen many patients with this problem respond to anti-Candida therapy. A clinical trial published in the *New England Journal of Medicine* by Professor S. Baker and Dr E.W. Rosenberg has supported this view (see Chapter 7). Anyone, therefore, who attends my clinic with psoriasis is going to be treated for candidiasis, as we know that psoriasis is nothing to do with allergy. This particular patient also had a history of excessive intestinal wind and bloating, pruritus ani, and sugar addiction.

As a precaution we first tried the standard elimination diet with, as expected, no obvious benefit. He was then changed immediately to the anti-Candida programme with increasing doses of Nystatin combined with the usual dict. Within eight weeks of starting this treatment his joints had become immensely freer. For the first time for years he could put his forehead on to his knees without any pain and he was no longer waking at night with pain. I emphasize he was taking no medication other than Nystatin. Further good news was that his psoriasis had greatly diminished and his only complaint then was that his constipation had not improved, but this frequently takes longer than a couple of months.

These last two cases illustrate the situation where the Candida problem was the cause of the whole situation. More commonly we see Candida complicating a food or chemical sensitivity problem and, if it is not dealt with, it makes the management of these problems unsatisfactory. Typical of this, and we have countless similar problems, was Wendy N.

When Wendy first attended the clinic she was 23 years old and had had rheumatoid arthritis since the age of 16. When I saw her the main problem joints were her knees and hands. The hands showed the typical severe ulnar deviation so characteristic of severe rheumatoid arthritis and the knees, apart from being painful and swollen, were fixed in a permanent position of flexion. She had taken a wide range of medications, including Chloroquine, Indocid, and Penicillamine. The last she had taken for over two years.

She improved a lot on our elimination diet and showed obvious severe reactions to wheat, rye, oats, tap water, monosodium glutamate, bananas, apples, pears, tomatoes, and grapefruit. Avoiding these foods produced a moderate improvement which was later enhanced considerably by the discovery of an insidious reaction to milk which she had initially thought to be innocuous. Skin tests were distinctly positive to house dust, dust-mite, etc. but neutralizing injections produced little benefit over and above that which had been obtained from the food identification. Measures to reduce the quantities of dust and mite in her immediate environment were instituted and produced some benefit.

The outstanding problem then with this patient was that neutralization therapy was not working at all well. She had inhaled allergies that were not responding, and many of her food sensitivities were unprotected by her neutralizing injections.

Problems with neutralization therapy are frequently related to untreated Candida problems. Candida toxin has been shown in the USA to decrease the level of T-lymphocytes which are the 'generals' of the immune system. Neutralization therapy is known not to work well in the presence of very depressed T-lymphocyte counts. Wendy was placed on the Phase 1 anti-Candida diet combined with Nystatin. In practice she did not tolerate Nystatin well, but had enormous improvement after being on caprylic acid for several weeks. The skin wheal responses, when she was tested intradermally, now showed up much better and good neutralizing levels were obtained. Soon she was able to cope with foods and inhalants that she had not managed before.

Her joints had now improved out of all recognition. The pain has virtually gone and the ulnar deviation in her hands is becoming straighter by the month. Her knees, which were fixed in a position of marked flexion, are now becoming straighter every month, helped in addition by exercises and hydrotherapy. This severely affected young lady with considerable joint destruction is nowadays over 80 per cent back to normal. The X-rays of her knees have improved enormously in appearance and the joint spaces now show over a quarter inch of extra space between the opposing bones. The radiologist in fact thought he was looking at the wrong X-rays as such improvement is virtually unheard of in the normal course of events.

Candidiasis treatment in this patient therefore produced marked benefit over and above that which was obtained by just isolating the specific food and inhalant sensitivities. We think that this is because the Candida problem is underlying these other problems. Without treating the candidiasis, the individual may well develop other food or inhalant sensitivities and in addition neutralization, which is essential in these complicated cases, may not succeed.

7 Psoriatic arthritis and ankylosing spondylitis

These two types of arthritis need, I think, some special consideration in addition to the general comments about other forms of arthritis.

Psoriatic arthritis

This name refers to the condition of those who have both psoriasis and arthritis. The arthritis is similar to rheumatoid arthritis, and 7 per cent of patients who have psoriasis have these arthritic complications; 20 per cent of patients who have a seronegative arthritis have psoriasis. The association is therefore so frequent as to suggest that whatever is causing the psoriasis in these patients may also be causing the arthritis. Experience indicates that this may indeed be so in some patients, but interestingly not in others.

Over the years I have been consulted by several patients with psoriasis in the hope that the 'allergy' approach might help them as it does with other skin disorders, such as eczema and urticaria. I did explore this possibility with several patients but drew a complete blank and then dissuaded any other patients from undergoing such investigation.

However, as mentioned in Chapter 6, I attended in 1981 the 15th Advanced Seminar of the Society for Clinical Ecology, held at Callaway Gardens, near Atlanta, Georgia. On the programme was the lecture by Dr Orion Truss on intestinal candidiasis which started my interest in that subject. One of the fascinating aspects of that lecture was the observation that he had seen several patients with psoriasis clear their skin problems spectacularly while on anti-Candida treatment regimes. Many slides showing major recovery from severe psoriasis were then demonstrated. Like all the best discoveries, this was a chance

observation that occurred when Dr Truss was treating patients
for other conditions who happened to have psoriasis at the same
time.

It was some months before another person with psoriasis
attended my clinic. I could hardly wait to use this new treatment,
and to my delight the patient responded dramatically within a
few months on large doses of Nystatin and the Candida diet.
Some 50 cases of psoriasis have now been treated in this manner
at the clinic, and without precisely counting I have the impression that about 80 per cent have done extremely well. This is of
course extremely important news to sufferers from psoriasis,
who account for between 1 and 2 per cent of the population of
the UK.

In the USA many physicians have successfully treated patients suffering from psoriasis in this way. One of the most
eminent is Professor William Rosenberg MD, Professor of
Dermatology in the Departments of Medicine and Pathology at
the University of Tennessee College of Medicine in Memphis.
Professor Rosenberg has now concluded that psoriasis is an
inherited fault in the body's antigen antibody response to foreign
organisms, especially Candida albicans. By way of further
explanation he has stated,

> *We think that psoriasis is a generalized inflammatory disorder
> initiated by microbial activation of the alternative complement
> pathway. The visible manifestations of psoriasis on the skin in this
> view occur partly because of microbial activators residing on the skin
> and partly as a result of the deposition in the skin of microbial
> products circulating in the bloodstream.*

Psoriasis runs in families and these families have been found to
lack certain genes called HLA genes (human leucocytic antigens). These genes produce appropriate defensive antibodies,
usually to invasion by Candida albicans, but if they are missing
the skin lesions of psoriasis result.

Apart from Nystatin, other anti-Candida drugs such as
Nizoral (ketoconazole) have also been used extensively. Sometimes Nizoral works better than Nystatin, presumably because it
is absorbed into the general circulation and does not remain
within the lumen of the gut like Nystatin. Nizoral does, though,
have a slight (1/10,000) risk of liver damage and has to be used
with care.

Dr Rosenberg has reported a 75 per cent success rate with

Nizoral given by mouth. He too has noticed additional improvement in some patients when using Nizoral cream in addition to the oral medication.

I would advise any physician who has a patient with psoriasis to try this approach. The treatment is simple. Increasing doses of Nystatin are given in accordance with the schedule I have suggested in Chapter 6. The patient is put on the Candida Phase 1 Diet. When substantial improvement has occurred, usually within two to three months, the Phase 2 foods can then be allowed. With further improvement, usually in another two to three months, the Phase 3 foods can also be returned to the patient's diet. In resistant cases Nizoral can be employed with careful monitoring of liver function by blood tests.

To return to arthritis we now need to ask, 'If psoriasis is caused by Candida albicans, is psoriatic arthritis also caused by the same organism?' The answer appears to be 'yes' in some cases, but in most cases, interestingly, the answer seems to be 'no'. In most cases of psoriatic arthritis, the arthritic component responds spectacularly to a hypo-allergenic diet within seven days, indicating that food allergy seems to be the main factor causing the disease. The skin problem in these patients has usually responded to the Candida treatment. In some other cases of psoriatic arthritis, however, there has been no benefit at all observed with a hypo-allergenic diet and both the psoriasis and the arthritis have responded to Candida therapy.

I will now describe two cases where food allergy seemed to cause the arthritic component of the problem and one case where candidiasis seemed to be responsible for both the joint and skin problem.

Stewart M., aged 31, was referred to me by a local consultant rheumatologist for investigation of his psoriatic arthritis. Stewart was a business development manager but was finding his occupation increasingly difficult to follow. He was a large man, weighing over 16 stone, and over 6ft 2inches in height. The joint problems had been present for four years, and at about the same time he started to notice psoriasis of his scalp and some psoriatic pitting of his finger nails. The arthritis was present in most of his joints, although the worst ones were his neck, back and the sternal area of his chest. Other problems occurred in his knees which were often badly swollen, his thumbs, fingers and right elbow. The joint problem had been helped to some extent by capsules of Indomethacin. Of interest to me, particularly in regard to the possibility of food sensitivity, was the fact that he had distinct fatigue, occasionally suffered from nocturnal sweats, and had generalized oedema which was not specifically related to his affected joints. His weight would fluctuate quite wildly at times and this symptom is very suggestive of food sensitivity.

As Stewart had a distinct psoriasis we immediately started him on Nystatin therapy, but concurrently he went on to our standard hypo-allergenic diet (see Chapter 9). On this diet there was initially a severe withdrawal reaction. On the first day Stewart had a severe headache for most of the day and this continued into the second day, when in addition he felt very low and depressed. On the second and third day there was considerable muscle pain (withdrawal myalgia) — a classic observation in such patients. The joints were particularly bad on the second and third day, but then slowly regressed so that by the seventh day there was marked improvement in all his joints, though he still had a fair amount of muscle pain. He had lost 11lb within the 6½ days and there was no change in the psoriasis.

Over the next two or three days the muscle pain disappeared and the joints improved further. When he introduced food back into his diet he had distinct reactions to pork, lamb, turkey, rabbit, potatoes, tea, rice, and corn. All these foods responded equally adversely when re-tested later. The reaction to lamb was particularly severe and obvious. Within 10 minutes he told me he had a headache; one hour later he was decidedly stiff and by four hours he was in total agony. As he said at the time, he changed within four hours from a young man to an old man. Later we used neutralization treatment to enable him to eat items such as corn and potatoes which were difficult for him to avoid, particularly in his business life. This worked perfectly satisfactorily.

Within two months of the initial consultation, I was able to write to his rheumatologist saying that he was currently taking no specific anti-arthritic drugs at all and that his joints were now almost entirely pain-free. He had lost 2 stone (28lb/13kg) in weight and his psoriasis had improved substantially. In addition he was feeling enormously better in himself, much brighter and much more clear-minded. His initial improvement maintained and increased over the subsequent four years and nowadays he is extremely well, with no evidence of arthritis or psoriasis.

Sheelagh C. was 41 years old when she first consulted me with both psoriasis and psoriatic arthritis. The psoriasis had been present since she was 19, but the joint pains and swelling had only been present for the preceding four years. Before consulting me she knew that citrus fruits and melon would make her joints decidedly worse, but avoiding them did not provide the whole answer. She noticed also that she was particularly fatigued when her joints were bad.

On the hypo-allergenic diet she suffered a moderately severe withdrawal reaction. On the evening of the first day she had a very nasty headache in the evening and vomited throughout the whole of the first night. The headache persisted most of the second day, but by the fourth day of this diet virtually all her joint pain had disappeared and she felt exceptionally well in herself. The foods she subsequently reacted to included wheat, corn, oats, rye, malt, potatoes, onions, garlic, orange, grapefruit, and spinach. She took neutralizing injections for these foods for the next few years and remained very well. Her psoriasis responded very satisfactorily to Nystatin and later to Nizoral.

The joints have remained well to the present day with a few very minor setbacks due to the fact that her neutralizing levels have changed. These slight hiccups have been corrected by retesting and giving her new neutralizing injections.

Deborah S., aged 13, consulted me with a history of psoriatic arthritis present for the preceding five years. The arthritis badly affected both her wrists, knees and left shoulder. There was slight pain in the ankles and toes. She had been under the care of one of the most famous rheumatologists in Britain and had been taking Naprosyn. There were patches of psoriasis on her neck and arms and she used Betnovate to help to control these. Her father had a distinct history of psoriasis itself, but had no joint complications.

Some patients with psoriatic arthritis seem to have a food sensitivity and some appear to be purely a candidiasis problem. In Deborah's case a hypo-allergenic diet extending over seven days produced no withdrawal effect and no improvement. We therefore changed our strategy and treated her for candidiasis, despite the fact that there was very little to indicate candidiasis in her history other than the fact that she had psoriasis. The only positive factors were a distinct sweet tooth and a history of constipation. We adopted our usual programme of increasing doses of Nystatin combined with the Phase 1 Candida Diet as described in Chapter 6. Within two months she had reached the 2 teaspoon dosage of Nystatin. Her joints were already feeling enormously better and the knees and hands were markedly less swollen. She told me that she was much more agile and was able to run again, the first time for years. The patches of psoriasis had regressed considerably and she has not needed to use Betnovate, the first time that this has happened for years. Improvement has continued up to the present day and she is now very well.

Ankylosing spondylitis

This is the form of arthritis in which the main problem occurs in the ligaments and tendons attached around the joints. The disease occurs mostly in the spine (poker back) and most commonly in the sacro-iliac joints at the base of the spine. There is a more extensive description of this condition in Chapter 8.

Although this is the third most common form of arthritis, we have only seen a handful of patients with this condition at our clinic, as opposed to over 1,000 with rheumatoid arthritis. There has been no published work linking this condition with allergy and this is probably the reason.

As we have seen so few cases, I feel less confident talking about this condition, but judging by the few we have seen it appears to respond to the same sort of approaches that we have used with rheumatoid arthritis, particularly the food allergy approach or the intestinal candidiasis approach.

One case was Joe E., mentioned in Chapter 1 as one of our three cases of arthritis. He had been diagnosed by a consultant rheumatologist as suffering from both rheumatoid arthritis and ankylosing spondylitis. He responded superbly to extensive allergy management, as detailed in the second chapter.

Another case was David J., who was aged 35 when he first consulted me. His joint problems had started when he was 22 years old but had increased relentlessly over the following 13 years. All his joints were involved, but his spine, shoulders, elbows, wrists, knees, and ankles were particularly bad. When I first saw him he took nearly 20 minutes to walk the 40 yards between my consulting room and his car. Other symptoms of note were wind and bloating, fatigue, pruritus ani, and a rash on his penis, possibly candidiasis, which had been present even before the joint problems had started.

As David was over 1 stone (14lb/6½kg) underweight when I first saw him, I was not anxious for him to go on to an elimination diet. Accordingly we skin-tested him with all the foods he normally ate using the intradermal provocative technique, and gave him neutralizing injections to those foods to which he was sensitive. Within two months his condition had changed out of all recognition and he had changed from a cripple to someone who went out most evenings and enjoyed himself. His only problems came when his neutralizing levels changed.

Later we realized that he had many features of candidiasis in his history, especially the pruritus ani and the rash on his penis. Going on to the Phase 1 Candida Diet and taking Capricin produced yet another quantum leap in his improvement. Nowadays he is at least 95 per cent better as compared with his original state when he saw us. When he keeps his carbohydrate level very low he is totally pain-free and has only the slightest residual stiffness. Perhaps a little more aggressive anti-Candida treatment will even get rid of this very slight symptomatology. Since having the Candida treatment his neutralizing levels have become totally static and he now no longer needs re-testing.

In November 1988, *The Independent* carried an account of work done by Dr Alan Ebringer, who is in charge of research into ankylosing spondylitis at the Department of Rheumatology at the Middlesex Hospital. He also works in the Department of Immunology at King's College, London. Dr Ebringer believes that this disease is a form of reactive arthritis caused initially by bacterial infection in the colon or rectum. The particular organism he is interested in is Klebsiella which, like Candida albicans, thrives on a diet rich in carbohydrates. The main plank of the treatment which he has used in more than 200 patients is to reduce drastically the carbohydrate content of the patient's diet. The majority of these patients have slowly but markedly improved. A drug called Salazopyrin can reduce levels of Klebsiella in the colon and this is usually given in conjunction with the diet.

It has been known for some time that 98 per cent of people who suffer from ankylosing spondylitis have the B27 tissue type. At King's College, screening tests were carried out to see whether any bacteria had a similarity to this tissue type. The experiment showed that the organisms which reacted with B27 were bowel bacteria such as Salmonella, Klebsiella, Shigella and Yersinia. Shigella and Yersinia cause diarrhoea, and it has been known for a long time that people who develop severe infection with these organisms can develop arthritis afterwards. Klebsiella, however, like Candida albicans, has always been regarded as a normal resident of the bowel.

Tests then performed by Dr Ebringer showed that patients with active ankylosing spondylitis had more Klebsiella in their stools than normal controls and more than in those patients whose disease was inactive. During active phases of the ankylosing spondylitis patients could be shown to have active antibodies to Klebsiella in their blood. Thus the immune system is precipitated by this bacteria into attacking by mistake the tissues of its own body, producing ankylosing spondylitis. Similar work has suggested that Proteus, an organism that normally causes urinary infections, may be linked with rheumatoid arthritis.

I think it is quite probable that a whole range of bacteria and yeasts could trigger this type of problem. The more we research these problems the more interested we become in the microflora of the lower digestive tract.

8 Different clinical types of arthritis

Arthritis is not a single disease entity, but consists of over 100 differing descriptive entities and syndromes. This type of problem dates back to antiquity, and prehistoric human remains have found to have signs of osteoarthritis. Some uncommon forms of arthritis such as viral and bacterial arthritis and rheumatic fever have well-known causes and effective treatments. The major causes of rheumatoid arthritis, osteoarthritis, ankylosing spondylitis, psoriatic arthritis and gout, are generally not well understood and form the main subject matter of this book.

Rheumatoid arthritis

This condition is characterized by pain, tenderness, swelling and stiffness of the joints, most commonly the smaller joints, especially those of the hands and wrists, although any joint can become affected. The condition is usually very long-standing and starts off as a pure inflammation. As this inflammation continues, joint destruction can gradually occur and the affected joints frequently become visibly deformed.

Rheumatoid arthritis mostly occurs between the ages of 25 and 50, but does also occur outside this age group. Females are affected three times more often than males.

The fact that the word 'rheumatoid' is used in the description of this disease suggests to many people that it may be brought on by cold and damp, but it is in fact just as common in hot countries. However, it is true to say that, althought it is no more common in cold, damp climates, it does tend to be more severe in such places.

Rheumatoid arthritis is usually connected with other symptoms occurring outside the joints. Fatigue, muscle pains and general malaise are very common. Inside the affected joints, the earliest change is one of swelling and congestion in the synovial membrane lining of the joint and the overlying connective tissue. Effusion of synovial fluid into the joint space accounts for the swelling of the joint. Later, thickening of the synovial membrame and fibrous adhesions across the joint spaces may occur. Muscles situated around the inflamed joints tend to deteriorate, partly through lack of use and partly because of involvement in the inflammatory process.

Rheumatoid arthritis can become complicated by pericarditis, vasculitis, pleurisy, peripheral neuritis, and various anaemias and other blood disorders. This collection of symptoms, a clinical picture, makes the diagnosis of rheumatoid arthritis likely and of course there are numerous variations on a theme. It is the blood tests, though, that really solidify the diagnosis.

The best-known test is the erythrocyte sedimentation rate (ESR). Erythrocytes are red blood cells which will settle in a tube of blood held vertically. As the cells settle they leave behind clear serum at the top of the tube which is easy to see and measure. Sedimentation rates are very much increased in, for example, rheumatoid arthritis but not in osteoarthritis. The ESR is quite a good index of severity. Many inflammatory conditions do lead to raised ESR so the test is suggestive but not totally diagnostic when applied to patients with joint pains.

Another test is that for rheumatoid factor, or the latex fixation test. This looks for the presence of rheumatoid factors or antibodies in the bloodstream. If the finding is positive these patients are referred to as seropositive. The outlook for these patients is worse than those who are seronegative. Patients, however, who are initially seronegative can later become seropositive.

Other tests can be performed on the fluid of the affected joints. The fluid can be obtained by aspiration with a small needle inserted into the joint. Tests such as antinuclear antibody (ANA), total complement test and immunoelectrophoresis tests all help to differentiate rheumatoid arthritis from non-specific arthritis and other similar conditions.

X-rays of the joints only really help to determine whether bones or cartilages have already been damaged by the disease. There are a number of other blood tests that are sometimes used as part of the evaluation or to monitor progress, but the ones I have just mentioned are the main ones.

Juvenile rheumatoid arthritis

This is a comparatively rare form of arthritis which affects children. There are several forms of the condition, the best known of which is Still's disease named after the physician, Frederick Still, of Great Ormond Street Hospital who initially named the condition. The outlook for these children is better than that for adults and 70 per cent will eventually recover spontaneously, usually around puberty.

Osteoarthritis

This is by far the commonest form of arthritis: five million people in Britain alone suffer from this condition. More properly, the condition is referred to as osteoarthrosis as the word osteoarthritis, finishing as it does with the term 'itis', implies that it is an inflammatory condition, whereas the clinical picture shows no inflammation. Usually it is regarded as a purely degenerative condition, but there is clearly an inflammatory side of the problem as it frequently responds beneficially to anti-inflammatory drugs. In fact the commonest treatment for osteoarthritis given by general practitioners is these particular drugs.

I was so imbued with the idea that this was a purely degenerative condition that I treated people with rheumatoid arthritis or non-specific arthritis for three years or so before a patient with osteoarthritis persuaded me to look at his condition as possibly being connected with allergenic or environmental factors. After witnessing great benefit in this patient I have treated many hundreds since with results similar to those obtained with the other major arthritises. I now consider that osteoarthritis is *not* a degenerative disorder in many people and have seen cases where the X-ray appearances of degeneration have markedly improved on follow-up after ecologic treatment. I now think that, although the condition is degenerative in that tissue degenerates, the degeneration is not just a matter in increasing age and wear and tear. I think that the 'degeneration' is very often caused by a poorly understood inflammatory process which in turn is influenced by allergic or environmental factors. Certainly we have seen cases where the X-ray appearances of joint narrowing and so on have improved after treatment to the point where the radiologist thought the X-rays had been mixed up with somebody else's.

In the normal course of events, the joint cartilages lose their elasticity and no longer provide a smooth seating for the bones of the joint. In bad cases the cartilage may wear away completely. At times the bones, unprotected now by cartilage, rub against each other and may polish their own surfaces. This may actually ease the joint pain but with the loss of cartilage there is a great decrease in mobility and flexibility.

One common feature of osteoarthritis is the hard knobs or nodes called Heberden nodes which most commonly develop around the finger joints. These knobs develop around the edge of the joints and are caused by the cartilage breaking up within the joint. The joints most susceptible to osteoarthritis are the big major joints of the body, such as the hips, knees, and spine. This contrasts with rheumatoid arthritis which most frequently affects the smaller, more peripheral joints such as the hands, wrists and feet.

Osteoarthritis is of course very common in people aged over 60, but it can affect many in their 20s and 30s.

Investigation of osteoarthritis reveals very many less positive features than rheumatoid arthritis. X-rays are the prime tool in such investigation and they can show the amount of deterioration in the joint mechanisms. The single most important finding here is how much the joint space has narrowed. Another interesting feature is the presence of osteophytes. These are little bony growths which develop when the cartilage has degenerated. The more numerous the osteophytes, the more cartilage has been lost. These findings are extremely common and occur in many people over 35 years old who have no sign of joint pain or stiffness. I noticed extensive osteophytes in my own thoracic spine 10 years ago when I had a routine chest X-ray. I have, however, never had any pain in that area. Blood tests reveal no abnormalities in osteoarthritis and serve only to distinguish it from those other forms of arthritis that do.

Ankylosing spondylitis

This is the next most common type of arthritis. It is the most common type of arthritis where the problem is situated at the point where ligaments and tendons attach to the joint bones as opposed to the problem being within the joint. The condition affects predominantly young and middle-aged men and in fact is present in men 10 times more commonly than women. It is similar to rheumatoid arthritis but in most cases it is quite a distinct problem on its own. In Chapter 1 the third case described, Joe E., had been diagnosed by an eminent rheumatologist as suffering from both rheumatoid arthritis and ankylosing spondylitis.

Spondylitis means 'inflammation of the joints of the spine'. Classically, pain occurs most often between the sacrum (the last bone of the spine) and the attached pelvis. The pain comes from the ligaments and tendons around that sacro-iliac joint. The classic sufferer has a rigid painful spine and difficulty in holding up his head when walking.

As in psoriatic arthritis, which will be discussed later, ankylosing spondylitis has a distinct genetic basis and it occurs in the relatives of sufferers 20 times more frequently than in the rest of the population. There are some people in the world, such as African negroes, where the condition is virtually unknown. Conversely American Indians, who may lead a similar non-civilized lifestyle, suffer the condition frequently. This would tend to confirm the importance of genetics in the predisposition to acquire the problem, but does not exclude the possibility that allergic or environmental factors may also be important.

Diagnosis of the condition is most helped by X-ray examination. X-rays will show classic changes in the sacro-iliac joints as long as the condition has been present for a year or so. Sedimentation rates are sometimes raised and sometimes not. A genetic test, the HLAB27 antigen blood test, shows if the patient has a genetic tendency to the disease, but it is quite possible to have a positive finding in this test and never develop the condition.

Certainly the development of iritis (an inflammation of the iris of the eye which makes it look red) in combination with chronic back pain should alert all to the possibility of this problem.

A variation of this type of problem is Reiter's disease. This is a rare condition and usually occurs in young men. It also has a genetic background but is usually triggered off by an infection, quite frequently gonorrhoea or another similar venereal disease. Certain forms of dysentery can also trigger the problem. The arthritic symptoms are usually combined with conjunctivitis and skin rashes.

Psoriatic arthritis

This seronegative inflammatory arthritis is found in patients with psoriasis. Psoriasis is a rather unpleasant skin disorder characterized by large scaling plaques. Sometimes the only outward sign of it is characteristic changes in the nails. This form or arthritis occurs in 7 per cent of patients who have psoriasis; and 20 per cent of all patients who have a seronegative arthritis have psoriasis, perhaps manifested only by the nail changes and sometimes overlooked because of this. Damage to the fingernails ranges from mild pitting to severe damage, thickening and discolouration.

The condition can affect any joint but usually involves only one or two. The joints near the finger tips are very likely to be affected. The problem in general is similar to rheumatoid arthritis but the joint damage is usually less severe. The ESR is only moderately raised and other specific tests for rheumatoid arthritis are negative. The conventional treatment of this condition is usually to use non-steroidal anti-inflammatory drugs and sometimes Gold injections. We find it responds well to the techniques described in Chapter 9.

Gout

The other name for this condition is crystal arthritis as tiny formations of minute crystals are found in the joint space, causing acute pain, swelling, and intense irritation. The crystals are caused by an excess of uric acid in the body and this in turn can be produced by a variety of factors. This is the one form of arthritis which has always been associated in the medical and public mind with dietary indiscretion, such as over-eating and over-drinking. The condition has been popularly associated with the rich and famous, particularly the aristocracy. There is a lovely passage in the book by Dr Colin H. Dong and Jane Banks entitled *New Hope for the Arthritic* (Granada, 1983):

> *A caricature of the gourmand King Henry VIII seen in comic strips is a picture description of gout that is worth 10,000 words. King Henry is shown as a fat, well-groomed monarch sitting on a great chair with his leg bandaged and with a big red inflamed toe exposed, resting on a foot-stool. In one hand he holds a large rib of beef and in the other hand a mug of ale.*

> *As a recent seminar in New Zealand I learned that when the native Maoris deserted their traditional fish and vegetable diet for the white man's one of beef, lamb, sweets and dairy products, they*

developed obesity, cardiovascular diseases and numerous cases of gout. This confirms the long-known fact that gout is a metabolic disease and that dietary transgression is one of the main causes.

The condition is, however, not confined to kings, lords and earls. It affects men rather than women in a ratio of 15:1. Sufferers are usually between the ages of 35 and 60 years old and the condition is to some extent genetically determined.

Patients usually have a high level of uric acid in their bloodstream for years; then possibly after a particularly rich meal an attack can occur, most commonly around the base of one of the big toes. This joint, the first metatarsophalangeal joint, is so commonly involved that when pain occurs in this joint it alerts all and sundry to the possibility of gout. The joint is not only painful and swollen but characteristically extremely tender to touch. Gout can, however, occur in almost any joint and a raised uric acid is what usually makes the diagnosis.

Apart from diet, a well-known cause of gout is diuretics. These drugs are used to get rid of excess water in the body and are commonly prescribed in cases of high blood pressure and heart failure.

Curiously I have been consulted by only a handful of patients with gout, despite the public association of this condition with dietary indiscretion. In most people the condition is intermittent and so elimination diets are a little problematic. Elimination diets are at their most convincing when used by those with continuous symptomatology. If the continuous symptomatology disappears after six days or so on such a diet all are suitably impressed. One patient who attended me a few years ago had mild continuous symptoms punctuated with severe attacks. All his symptoms disappeared entirely on the elimination diet and returned after three separate consumptions of butter taken at weekly intervals. The butter had the yellowing agent, tartrazine, present and since avoiding this item he has had no further recurrence in the past seven years. Other patients with gout have their own individualized dietary problems. It is not just caused by port!

Systemic lupus erythematosus

This condition resembles rheumatoid arthritis and can affect any joint. It is a multi-system connective tissue disorder characterized by the presence of numerous auto-antibodies, circulating immune complexes and very widespread immunologically determined tissue damage.

It usually affects young women and has distinct genetic tendencies. It is know to be induced by many separate drugs and also by sunlight. It is nevertheless considered to be mostly an auto-immune condition, a view with which I disagree as I have seen a number of patients respond to allergy and environmental management. Furthermore, if the condition were solely auto-immunity then drugs surely would not cause it. The most well-known feature of this condition is the red rash which spreads across the nose and cheek, looking in shape rather like a butterfly. I have a couple of patients where this rash has disappeared after sorting out their food allergies.

Polymyalgia rheumatica

Polymyalgia rheumatica is a condition that should be mentioned here. Predominantly it is a muscle disorder but the joints frequently become involved. It affects mostly the hips and shoulders of individuals over 50 years old. It is diagnosed by the presence of distinct muscle pain and tenderness and a markedly raised ESR.

The first polymyalgia rheumatic sufferer I ever saw managed from an ecological point of view was a patient of Dr Richard Mackarness at Basingstoke. This patient had an extremely severe form of the condition and she responded brilliantly to Dr Mackarness's treatment. At the time I was incredibly impressed by this patient's progress as she had seen many eminent physicians before without any benefit at all. Her continued complete recovery was one of the major reasons why I became interested in this subject.

Other forms of arthritis

There are other forms of arthritis, mostly of an acute nature, which are caused by micro-organisms and are already well understood and treated. They having nothing to do with the main subject matter of this book but are included here in the interests of completeness.

Viral arthritis

This can be caused by viruses such as rubella (German measles). The joints become painful and swollen but the pain disappears in a few weeks without any specific treatment.

Septic (bacterial) arthritis

This condition usually has a sudden and spectacular onset with severe joint pain and swelling, a high fever and malaise. It is caused by bacteria such as Staphylococci, Streptococci and Haemophilus influenzae, sometimes introduced by medical procedures. It is particularly likely to occur in people already suffering from rheumatoid arthritis or diabetes. Antibiotic treatment and possible joint drainage are effective treatments and the condition normally does not create any long-term problems.

Rheumatic fever

This condition usually follows a throat infection caused by Streptococci. Widespread use of antibiotics for such infections has probably led to a huge decrease in the incidence of this disease.

It usually affects children and the pains flit from one joint to another. The joints are swollen, painful and hot, and accompanied by a fever. The condition responds well to rest and Penicillin but about 50 per cent of sufferers may develop some problem with the valves of their heart, particularly the mitral valves.

9 The elimination diet

An elimination diet is one of the most useful tools in medicine. It is cheap and, as long as it is done sensibly, perfectly safe. Ideally, such a diet should be conducted under the care and guidance of a physician experienced in its use. However, in the UK at the moment there are only a few specialized hospital departments and a number of private clinics that are set up to provide this type of service. Some of the private clinics are quite reasonable but they are, even so, beyond the purse of many people.

It is partly for this reason that I have decided to include a step-by-step guide telling you how to go through an elimination diet without actually attending a clinic. Another reason is that this book is also written for physicians and nutritionists interested in this approach, and these details will give them practical guidance in dealing with their patients.

As one might expect, some sufferers find an elimination diet very acceptable, very easy to follow and very easy to assess. These people find that there is an enormous reduction, often over 90 per cent, in their arthritic symptoms after six to eight days on a low-risk diet. They then start reintroducing foods into their diet and notice sharp reactions to about three or four foods only. If these foods are reasonably easy to avoid they do so, and frequently they have virtually no more problems with arthritis for the rest of their lives.

Others may find that their symptoms clear very well after six to eight days on the diet, but seem to react to a large number of foods, often as many as 15–20 separate items. When I was first involved with this subject I found it difficult to accept that people could react to so many different foods, but after many years and much re-testing of foods I consider that most of these observations have been quite genuine. Sufferers do not want to react adversely, particularly to their favourite foods, and there is probably more of a tendency to disregard minor reactions to favourite foods than to invent reactions that don't exist.

The most difficult cases are a small minority who have incredibly slow and insidious reactions to foods. Such people may take 12–24 hours to react to a food like milk, which most people will react to in less than five hours. If, in addition, they react to a large number of foods, then an elimination diet can be an extremely difficult, frustrating, and highly unsatisfactory procedure. They may go for days or weeks trying to find a few foods they appear to be all right with. Such people can, if they are not careful, run themselves into considerable nutritional difficulties, and when they relate their experience to physicians who are not familiar with the advantages and pitfalls of elimination diets, the physicians may be somewhat dismayed at what they have done and adopt an extremely negative attitude to the whole concept.

Those whose symptoms clear nicely after the first few days of the Stage I diet, but who find themselves apparently reacting to a very large number of foods, should abandon the elimination diet and have their allergies sorted out by intradermal provocative skin testing. Certainly this would apply to someone reacting to four or five or more of the first six foods that are tried. My only reservations regarding the wisdom of detailing an elimination diet in this book concerns this very point. I know how determined some people become once they have seen their arthritic symptoms improve without the benefit of drugs on the first stage of this diet.

Preparation

As food allergy is involved in at least 85 per cent of sufferers from arthritis, it is worth while for *all arthritis sufferers* to try such a diet. It is, nevertheless, advisable to do some self assessment before you begin the diet.

1.   Is there a high chance that I have a food allergy?

Food allergy questionnaire   *Point Score*
1. **Fatigue**
     Slight   10
     Moderate   20
     Severe   30

2. **Obesity**
    (Weight able to fluctuate by 4 lb or more
    within a day)   20
    In addition:
    1 stone overweight   5
    2 stone overweight   10
    3 stone or more overweight   15

3. **Swelling and puffiness of face,
    ankles or fingers**
    (Not the swelling specifically related to
    arthritically inflamed joints)
    Slight swelling   10
    Moderate swelling   20
    Bad to the extent of needing to take
    diuretics (water pills)   30

4. **Bouts of sweating for no obvious cause**   20
    (For example, waking up at night feeling hot
    and sweaty. This does not include menopausal
    sweats unless they have been present for
    five years or more.)

5. **Bouts of your heart beating fast**
    Very occasionally   10
    Frequent   20

6. **Any history of known food intolerance
    causing any symptoms**
    One food known   10
    Several foods   20

7. **Does the consumption of alcohol make
    your joints worse the following morning?**
    Yes   30

8. **Any history of dependence, craving for,
    or addiction to such foods as:**
    Bread
    Sugar
    Chocolate   15
    Milk
    Coffee
    Tea

9. **A history of any other condition known to be connected with food allergy, such as:**
   Migraine
   Severe headaches
   Irritable bowel syndrome
   Eczema
   Urticaria $\left.\right\}$ 15
   Depression
   Asthma
   Myalgia (aching muscles)

As can be seen, it is possible to score 215 points on this questionnaire, but the highest I have seen in clinical practice would be around 180 points. Most people who prove to have food allergy underlying their arthritis would have a score of around 50 points. Anyone with a score of higher than 70 could feel very confident that food allergy was their problem.

A symptom score system like this can easily be criticized as it is fairly subjective in some areas. For example, one person may consider their fatigue to be moderate, whereas another may consider the same fatigue to be severe. Some of the other questions, however, can only invite a straight 'yes' or 'no' response. Another criticism of this questionnaire might be the reaction that most rheumatoid arthritis sufferers are known to suffer fatigue in any case. I would agree with this, but the reason they do so, in my view, is that most of them have food allergy and fatigue as the hallmark of food allergy. Fatigue normally disappears on elimination diets after the first few days.

Chemical sensitivity

Chemical sensitivity can complicate the picture in some sufferers from arthritis. In my experience, the biggest single problem is natural gas sensitivity. People can be sensitive to petrol fumes, diesel fumes, paint fumes, perfumes, bleaches, disinfectants, etc., but in most cases the contact is comparatively transitory and as such is relatively unimportant.

Experience shows that those with chemical sensitivity tend to know petrol or diesel fumes upset them, but are unaware of the fact that gas from gas cookers, gas central heating boilers, or gas water heaters permeate through the whole house and can take days of ventilation to eradicate. Those who know that they have headaches, distinct nausea or fatigue from contact with petrol fumes, diesel fumes, paint fumes, cigarette smoke, nail varnish, disinfectants and so on should strongly consider turning off all gas utilities before they start their elimination diet. In the winter months this can be a fairly traumatic idea, particularly as the house should be ventilated as well as the utilities being turned off at the mains. In these circumstances it is usually a good idea to wait until the weather is warm before embarking on the procedure. The gas utilities should be turned off for about five days before beginning the diet if there is a strong suspicion of gas sensitivity. Cheap electric hobs or microwave cookers can be used temporarily to substitute for gas cooking.

Sufferers with access to an allergy clinic involved in the clinical ecology approach can have intradermal skin tests with a natural gas exhaust reagent, and also with synthetic ethanol. Distinctly positive tests with these reagents would confirm gas sensitivity. Some people notice that they are obviously worse joint-wise when their gas utilities are on and are better when they are away from them, as when on holiday in a hot, dry climate. Such people must definitely turn their gas off before they begin an elimination diet, as it will undoubtedly confuse the results enormously.

Rarely, sufferers may be sensitive to formaldehyde, or perhaps phenol. Formaldehyde is used for cavity wall insulation and in plaster board, and is generally widely involved in the basic construction of many modern homes. It is, therefore, very difficult to avoid, short of staying in an environmental control unit or a house built before modern building materials were available.

Phenol is the gas given off by plastics. The softer the plastic the more phenol is produced. Modern houses have a lot of plastic in their construction and decoration and it can be very expensive to remove. Skin-testing is again helpful in these cases, which are fortunately not very frequent in my experience.

Other inhaled allergies

Allergies to house dust/house dust mite and moulds can be very important in arthritis. These problems rarely occur on their own, but I have seen them very frequently existing in addition to the food sensitivity problem. What is often observed in those who are about 70 per cent improved on the diet is that they are skin-tested to house dust/house dust mite/moulds, found positive, and when neutralizing injections are administered they then have a further quantum improvement, maybe to 95 per cent improved.

If you are doing an elimination diet on your own, I can only say that you should be aware that this possibility exists, particularly if you have noticed that holidays in hot dry countries of the Mediterranean, such as Spain or Greece, have resulted in temporary improvement of your arthritis (there is little house dust mite or mould in those countries).

You have, therefore, at this point prepared yourselves for the elimination diet. The higher the score on the food allergy scoring sheet the higher the probability that the elimination diet will yield a positive result in terms of symptom relief within a period of six to eight days. Should there be a distinct chemical problem, the gas should be turned off. Evidence of dust/mite or other inhalant sensitivity should alert you to the possibility of such complications, which perhaps are best dealt with during the elimination diet if things are not going too well.

It is important for a patient to select a good time to do an elimination diet, as it is a very anti-social procedure. Eating out, eating at other people's houses and so forth are virtually impossible in the first two or three weeks of this procedure. There is in fact some difficulty but not impossibility, in this respect for the whole eight weeks duration (approx.) of the elimination diet. It is also a good idea to choose a time when maximum support can be obtained from people who are close to you and are concerned about the problem you are having with your arthritis.

Drugs

Perhaps the biggest single problem on starting an elimination diet is the fact that, usually, ongoing drugs have to be discontinued while you are on the diet. The reason for this is that virtually all anti-arthritic drugs contain foodstuffs in the matrix of the tablets. The standard way in which a pharmaceutical company will make up a tablet is to pour cornflour or lactose (from milk) into a mould and then add the active chemical ingredient. Corn is the second commonest food allergy, and milk is the third. Normally a little morsel of cornflour or lactose in tablets does not matter, as you are eating these foods several times a day already in other forms, but when you are in the first stage of an elimination diet it does matter. Even a small amount of a food to which are are allergic can have a profound effect. If you are corn-allergic and are consuming small lumps of corn starch in the form of tablets in the first stage of your elimination diet, your symptoms will probably not clear and you will consider your problem not to be food allergy.

To give you some examples:
Brufen contains maize starch and sugar
Feldene contains lactose and corn starch
Indocid (Indomethacin) contains sugars and maize starch
Enteric-coated Deltacortril contains sugar, corn starch and lactose
Penicillamine contains maize starch.
✓ Naprosyn, in contrast, contains no food excipients at all.

Medications which are satisfactory would include soluble aspirin and soluble Prednisolone (Predsol made by Glaxo).

As most people know, Cortisone, either in the form of Prednisolone, Betnesol or whatever, must *NEVER* suddenly be discontinued. When Cortisone has been taken over a long period, the adrenal glands become suppressed by the Cortisone present artificially in the bloodstream. If this Cortisone is suddenly discontinued, then the individual has virtually no Cortisone with which to deal with all the normal physical stresses of everyday life. This can lead to very dire consequences if any major stress is encountered. For patients attending my clinic we substitute Prednesol, which contains no foodstuffs, for other forms of Cortisone with their existing physician's agreement.

Patients who have been on oral Prednisolone for several years often respond poorly to food allergy elimination procedures. It seems as if the Cortisone has fossilized their immune systems and the arthritis may become irreversible. Those who are on Cortisone should not attempt an elimination diet without close medical supervision. Other 'disease modifying drugs' such as Penicillamine and Gold should only be ceased under the supervision of the consultant rheumatologist who is conducting the case.

The non-steroidal anti-inflammatory drugs, such as In-domethacin, Feldene, Naprosyn and Brufen, can be stopped without any great problems. There will be, though, more pain than usual in the first part of the elimination diet, partly because of the withdrawal effect already described, and partly because the 'drug crutch' has been removed. By about day 5 this, hopefully, will not matter as the arthritis should be improving substantially by then. For those who can tolerate it, soluble aspirin is a reasonably satisfactory crutch for the first few days of the diet should it be needed.

Aside from drugs used to relieve or control arthritis, some sufferers may be taking other drugs, such as the contraceptive pill, sleeping tablets, and blood pressure tablets. The contraceptive pill contains cornflour etc., as do the other pills. Obviously the contraceptive pill must be discontinued at the end of a specific reproductive cycle and mechanical means of contraception used temporarily during the elimination procedure.

Sleeping tablets or capsules are a great problem for some. People often become very dependent on them and cannot sleep without them. One possible solution is a switch to Temazepam (Normison) temporarily, as this contains no foodstuff.

Blood pressure pills also have to be discontinued and your GP should be told of this. I have never seen anyone's blood pressure rise on the first stage of the diet, and very frequently it goes down, despite the withdrawal of the blood pressure pills. The reason for this is that many blood pressure problems are ultimately caused by food sensitivity.

The elimination diet

Having sorted out the drug problem, we can now come to the diet itself. An elimination diet starts with a low-risk allergy diet called by some an oligo-antigenic diet. Such a diet consists of a handful of foods which you rarely eat and which have a known low risk of allergy. These foods are used simply for you to 'keep the wolf from the door' while you avoid all the likely incriminatory foods. For arthritis the foods I would most frequently start with are as follows:

cod
trout
mackerel
pears
avocado pears
parsnips
turnips
swedes (rutabaga)
sweet potatoes (yams)
celery

marrow
courgettes (zucchini)
carrots
peaches (only when available fresh)

For cooking you can use sunflower oil or safflower oil, whichever you use less frequently.

If you eat any of the above list more frequently than two times a week, that food should be omitted from the diet.

Any strict vegetarian who wishes to do this diet would of course have to omit the fish, but could possibly add bamboo shoots to make the diet a little less restrictive.

The only liquid which is allowed on the diet is one of the bottled spring waters, such as Malvern water, Evian, Perrier, Volvic, Highland Spring, etc. It does not appear to matter whether the water is still or sparkling and this can be left to personal taste. Should you wish to liquidize the carrots, pears or peaches with the spring water and make a vegetable or fruit juice, this would of course be quite acceptable.

Pure sea salt can be used for flavouring the food.

It is to be emphasized that cigarette smoking must be totally discontinued as soon as you go on to the elimination diet for the reasons mentioned in Chapter 4. As explained in this chapter, generally it is easier than usual for you to discontinue smoking while on a low-risk allergenic diet.

There remain three further pieces of advice which you should follow:

• Sodium bicarbonate solution should be substituted for toothpaste, as various components of toothpaste can be absorbed under the tongue and cause problems.

• Licking stamps and envelopes can cause problems as the glue contains corn and several chemicals.

• A large dose of Epsom salts should be taken on the first morning of the elimination diet to eliminate foods consumed on the days preceding the diet. Two teaspoons of Epsom salts are adequate for most adults and one teaspoon for children over 5 years old. The Epsom salts should be dissolved in about ¼ pint of spring water.

It is only to be emphasized that the above list of foods are the *ONLY* foods that you can eat on Stage I of this diet. There is, therefore, no tea, no coffee, no bread, no milk, no sugar, no eggs, etc. British people find that breakfast is the most strange meal to have to cope with using these restrictions. For those who just wish to have a snack, some pears, avocado pears, celery, carrots, or peaches should suffice. There is, however, no reason why you should not have a cooked breakfast with one of the fishes combined with one of the vegetables. The main meals of the day can contain a large quantity of fish with plenty of root vegetables and marrow, finishing with some fruit.

This is, therefore, a strange diet. Some people with very positive attitudes quite enjoy it and like the challenge it presents to them. If they also find their arthritic symptoms rapidly disappearing, then the whole procedure is quite joyful.

Others can find the diet very trying. They feel upset that they cannot eat their bread, drink their tea, etc. They sometimes complain they cannot face eating foods other than what they are used to eating every day of their lives. They have what a close colleague of mine, Dr Jonathon Maberly, has termed 'grief reaction' for their 'lost foods'. Amazingly, such patients can arrive on the seventh day of the elimination diet showing enormous or total improvement in their arthritis and still be quite unhappy because their diet is so restricted. They do not appear to appreciate the enormity of the fact that their symptoms have gone.

What happens on Stage I

At this point it is important to recall the whole concept of masking which was described in detail in Chapter 2. When you go on to a few safe foods you should, if you have a masked food allergy, feel distinctly worse for the first three or four days of the Stage I diet. You are no longer obtaining the temporary lift that further doses of the allergenic food normally give you. You are, therefore, worse on the first few days of going on to this diet for the same reasons that the alcoholic is worse when or or she stops taking alcohol.

Classically the afternoon/evening of the first day usually sees a distinct worsening of the joint pains. In those who have discontinued their daily anti-inflammatory or analgesic (pain-killing) drugs this may seem quite normal and to be expected. However, it also occurs in those who have not been taking drugs before the start of the diet. Those who have discontinued drugs may be suffering, therefore, for two reasons: (1) the drug discontinuation; and (2) the food withdrawal. The afternoon and evening of the first day of the diet are frequently accompanied by a severe headache if you are in any way prone to these. Should you normally suffer from migraines, that can virtually be guaranteed to occur on the first day.

The second day of the diet is also usually a very bad day. The joint pains are quite severe and fatigue is often a marked feature. There may be some headache left over from the first day and about 50 per cent of patients spend most of the second day in bed. At my clinic we often have a 'second-day phone call' from concerned relatives who may not understand the logic of the withdrawal phenomenon.

The third day of the diet is sometimes as bad as the second day, and by now there may be depression coming into the clinical picture. Some people may, however, notice a small reduction in joint swelling and pain by this day.

However, the third day very frequently marks the onset of *withdrawal myalgia*, which is one of the classic features of the allergy withdrawal syndrome. Typically, muscle aches and pains (as opposed to joint aches and pains) occur in the lower back, buttocks, and thighs. Sometimes these pains occur in other major muscle groups, such as the shoulders, arms, neck, and lower legs. These pains are often quite severe on days 3, 4, and 5. I have had many patients tell me that on day 5 their joint pains have improved greatly, but they feel crippled by the muscle pain which they do not normally experience. These muscle pains usually ease on days 6 and 7, although they occasionally go on until days 8 or 9. These muscle pains are usually nothing to worry about.

The overriding concern in the latter part of the elimination diet is, however, to observe a large decrease in joint pain, swelling, and stiffness. This is what ultimately shows that one is on the right lines with a particular individual. Sometimes the improvement in the joints is obvious as early as the fourth day, but often little benefit will occur jointwise until day 6.

The end of stage I – evaluation day 7

This is the time to really take stock of what has happened since the start of the diet. I always see patients under my care on this day. What I am predominantly concerned about on this day is how the patient feels jointwise. Those whose problems are exclusively food sensitivity often rate themselves 80–90 per cent improved on this day. Usually they are better than they would normally be with the presence of drugs in their bloodstream.

If such an improvement has occurred, particularly with a characteristic story of withdrawal symptoms on the first three days of the diet, I am happy that we are dealing with a food allergy. The contrast of the worst two or three days the patient has recently experienced followed two days later by the best two days is usually so marked that it is difficult to imagine it has occurred by chance.

Some people show virtually no withdrawal reaction at all. Their symptoms are the same as usual on days 1–3, generally followed by a gradual improvement on days 4, 5 and 6. I have no idea why this should occur, as they frequently turn out to have just the same sort of food allergies as those who suffer the classic withdrawal symptoms.

Another odd pattern I sometimes see is someone who follows the classic pattern until day 6. Expecting to arise better than ever on day 7, they awake to find their joint pain has occurred again in full force.

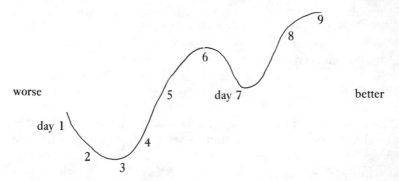

Figure 2   Withdrawal pattern followed by echo response

Happily, these pains normally go away about 36 hours later. Sometimes this phenomenon, which I call an 'echo effect', occurs a bit later on the evening of the seventh day after testing the first food on Stage II. The individual will properly ascribe the recurrence of symptoms to that food, but on re-trial a week later usually no reaction occurs. Why this echo effect occurs I have no idea, but similar things occur in classic immunology and there may soon be a logical explanation for it.

If, therefore, there is the satisfactory outcome of distinctly diminished joint paints, swelling, and possibly stiffness, you can now proceed into the second stage in which you slowly reintroduce foods that have a relatively low risk of allergy into the diet.

In my experience of about 2,000 patients with arthritis of any type, about 85 per cent will be showing definite benefit by day 7 or possibly day 8 of the diet. Let us now consider the 15 per cent (approx.) who do not. They will normally show the following reaction:

- a flat curve of response with no worsening initially in the first few days of the diet and no improvement towards the end. They are not normally, I consider, food allergic. Some of them may be suffering exclusively from inhaled allergy or possibly reacting to the yeasts in the flora of their gut. A few cases of rheumatoid arthritis related to zinc deficiency have been described and this may be the cause in some of these patients. Some will reveal no such factors and currently may have to be given up from the allergy/nutritional point of view and return to conventional suppressive medication.

- a withdrawal reaction initially, but then no distinct improvement. The withdrawal is due to the sudden cessation of the food to which they are sensitive. The lack of improvement may be due to the fact that they are sensitive to something on the low-risk diet. The most likely items would be the fish and a few more days on this diet omitting the fish has in some people cleared the symptoms.

Stage II

The prime object of this stage is to expand the diet as quickly as possible. To that end you should select, especially in the first three or four days, foods which are unlikely to give adverse reactions. There then follow foods which are generally desirable, but have only a moderate risk of allergy. A suggested order of introduction follows. It is advisable to stick to this rigidly, as the safer foods are introduced earlier, and members of similar food families are separated by four days. This avoid the possibility of false negative responses due to cross-reactivity within specific food families. Two foods are included for each day, starting with one food on the evening of day 7 after the seventh-day evaluation. One food should be tested in the morning at breakfast time and one in the evening, thus allowing at least nine or ten hours between tests. This should be adequate time for reaction to these foods to develop. Lunchtime is limited to those foods that were on Stage I or which have already been passed as safe on Stage II. It does not matter on any particular day which of the two foods are tested in the morning and which in the evening.

Stage II order of food reintroduction

Day 7	(evening) broccoli
Day 8	runner beans
	chicken
Day 9	tomatoes
	lamb (lamp chops or roast lamb)
Day 10	brown rice
	bananas
Day 11	tap water
	black tea (whichever tea you normally consume)
Day 12	cow's milk (whole milk as delivered by the milkman)
	grapes
Day 13	apples
	pork
Day 14	potatoes
	leeks
Day 15	eggs
	melon
Day 16	beef
	yeast (brewer's yeast – 2 teaspoons)
Day 17	butter
	cabbage

In the event of one of the foods being unavailable, natural dates obtained from a health food shop (not in presentation boxes) or fresh pineapple can be substituted wherever you wish.

When testing a food, the most important thing to watch for is the recurrence of arthritic symptoms. However, if headache, fatigue or other symptoms occur, it is still sensible to regard this as a reaction and drop the food from the diet, at least for the time being. Symptoms most commonly occur within four to five hours, but nine or ten hours exist between tests to accommodate those who tend to react slowly.

Reactions to food vary largely in intensity, like everything in life. The big bad reactions are extremely obvious to all patients. Before the reaction occurs, the joints are probably feeling very good, but within two to three hours of eating the allergic food you feel 'crippled'. The contrast of feeling so good followed within a few hours by so bad is obvious. Other reactions are moderately obvious, but inevitably the situation sometimes arises when you are not sure. What usually happens is something like this.

You consume a food at 8.00 a.m. Later that morning you do something moderately energetic like gardening, heavy house-work or shopping, and the joints flare mildly in the afternoon. Is this a mild reaction to the food or a response to the exercise? Certainly in the early days of the elimination diet there will be residual inflammation in the joints, which can be stirred up by mild exercise. There is only one way out of this dilemma, and that is to re-test the food. The ultimate saving grace of elimination diets is the ability to re-test.

On the day of the re-test you must make sure that there are no confusing variables, such as heavy exercise, to confuse the issue again. However, the most important rule to obey is NEVER RE-TEST A FOOD WITHIN FIVE DAYS OF THE ORIGINAL TEST. The only time an immediate reaction to a food occurs is when it has been omitted from the diet for a minimum of five days. If it is omitted for a shorter period than this, a reaction will occur, but it will be delayed and possibly not associated with that food. Thus the two major rules of food testing are:

- if in doubt about a food reaction, leave the food out of the diet.
- never re-test a food in less than five days from the original test.

When a reaction to a food occurs, within a few hours all the old pain, swelling, and stiffness will flood back. This reaction can last anything from about 12 hours to four or five days, and during this time no further testing can be accomplished. You must therefore restrict yourself to those foods already found to be safe until the symptoms pass. This of course slows up the testing programme and all the timing of reintroducing foods on certain days changes. To speed up the clearing of a reaction the following mixture is strongly recommended:

2 teaspoons of sodium bicarbonate
1 teaspoon of potassium bicarbonate

These two bicarbonates are placed in ¼ pint (140 ml) of hot water and stirred until dissolved. The sodium bicarbonate is ordinary bicarbonate of soda, which is obtainable at any chemist or supermarket. The potassium bicarbonate can be quite difficult to obtain. However, your chemist should be able to get it from a wholesaler.

The mixture is pretty revolting to take and most people prefer to swallow it with one gulp. It usually does two things:

- It gives you a bowel movement and the allergic food tends to be eliminated from the intestines. Clearly the faster this occurs, the better.
- Food reactions are accompanied by a reactionary acidosis: all your body fluids become slightly more acid, and this indirectly causes many of the symptoms. A large dose of alkali corrects this situation to some extent.

This medication, therefore, acts in two separate and complementary ways. A single dose of the bicarbonate mixture will normally halve the reaction time. If you can face a further dose it can be taken four to six hours later to further help the reaction to subside. The time for you to restart testing is when the symptoms from the preceding reaction have subsided.

At the end of Stage II there should be a general review of what has occurred. Hopefully there will have been a substantial improvement in the symptoms by the end of Stage I, followed by a maintenance of that improvement for most of Stage II. Individuals who have only two or three food sensitivities may negotiate the whole of Stage II with no reaction at all.

Two main questions are worth asking at this point. The most important is: how much improvement has been obtained up to this point? In other words, except when you have been reacting to a food on Stage II, are you 30 per cent better, 50 per cent better, 70 per cent or 90 per cent? If you are something like 90 per cent improved by the end of Stage II (between reactions), then your problems are almost certainly exclusively food allergy. The remaining 10 per cent improvement will probably occur naturally within the next month or so as the residual inflammation in the joints subsides.

If you are only 30–70 per cent improved, there is probably an inhaled component to your problems. This may be either a chemical problem such as gas, or one of the common inhaled allergens such as house dust, house dust mite, moulds, or animal danders. These usually need a competent allergist familiar with this approach to sort out (see appropriate chapters).

There are 21 foods on Stage II. Quite a lot of people will react to five or six of these foods and such individuals will normally end up with about 12–16 food allergies by the end of Stage IV. These people will eventually almost certainly need neutralization therapy to enable them to eat relatively normally in the long run. Anyone reacting to something like 15 or more of the 21 foods should immediately resort to the intradermal skin testing and neutralization approach. Should there be a delay before you can obtain this type of help, you should resume a normal diet plus your original drugs in the intervening time.

Stage III

You can now embark on this stage which contains many common food allergens, including the cereals, which need special consideration in their testing. Cereals, especially wheat, are very slowly absorbed and most frequently take 36 hours to react. I have seen some patients even take over two days to react to wheat and this, therefore, must be taken into account.

Day 18   ground coffee
                          oranges

Days 19, 20 & 21   wheat
                          Test either as wholewheat macaroni, wholewheat spaghetti or pure shredded wheat. Shredded wheat is probably the best test, but it is difficult to consume if milk has not been found to be satisfactory on the last stage. The pure wheat should be eaten at all meals on these three days (plus all safe foods). The reaction to this foodstuff is not only slow to materialize, but if it occurs it is very slow to eradicate. I have seen some patients take four to five days before they feel well again.

Day 22   wholemeal bread
                          This should only be tested if both the wheat test and the yeast test are satisfactory. Try wholemeal bread at each meal for this day.

Day 23	onion
	spinach

Day 24   cane sugar

This is a Jamaican, Trinidad or other West Indian demerara sugar. Muscovado is also satisfactory. Two teaspoons of cane sugar should be taken three times a day for one full day.

Day 25   mushrooms

peanuts

The peanuts should be obtained loose from a health food shop. Do not use the packeted variety, which have other additions.

Day 26   beet sugar

This is retailed under the name of Silver Spoon in the UK and marketed by the British Sugar Corporation. Usually it is pure beet sugar but sometimes, if the beet sugar crop is inadequate in quantity, there can be a little cane sugar added to it as well. Allergies to cane sugar and beet sugar are quite separate, as they come from totally different plants. Please note that Tate & Lyle sugar has both cane sugar and beet sugar in most samples. Spend one day on testing beet sugar, taking two teaspoons at each meal.

Day 27 & 28   corn

This very commonly consumed food should be tested in two forms: (1) corn on the cob, and (2) pure glucose powder. Glucose retailed in Britain is nearly always made from corn, although most retail chemists are unaware of this. Start each meal with corn on the cob (or loose) and finish the meal with two teaspoons of glucose. Take both forms of corn at each meal for two full days. Some people appear to react more obviously to one form of corn and some to the other. Either way, the reaction is to corn. Reactions to corn are slow but usually not

quite as slow as wheat and I have not seen
them starting longer than 48 hours after
commencing this test.

Day 29   lettuce
                          soya beans
                              Soy is very important. It is present in
                              soya-bean oil (vegetable oils), soya-bean
                              flour, etc. One way or another it is pre-
                              sent in a huge range of manufactured
                              foods.

Day 30   Cheddar cheese
                          bacon (if pork is satisfactory)
                              When testing for bacon one is in fact
                              testing for the nitrites and nitrate chemic-
                              als that are present in bacon. Check there
                              is no sugar mentioned on the packet.

End of Stage III assessment

Most people will have reacted to at least one food by now. The
Western diet is predominantly based on wheat, corn, cane sugar,
beet sugar, yeast, milk, eggs, soy, and potatoes. These main
foods have not all been tested and usually at this point you will
have a shrewd idea of your problems. Otherwise, the comments
I made on the Stage II assessment equally apply at this stage.

Stage IV

The object of Stage IV is to tidy up all the loose ends. If you
notice that your reaction to Stage II foods started within five
hours, then three foods a day can now be tested (except for the
remaining cereals). If not, continue on two foods a day.

Day 31   white bread (do not test if you are
                          allergic to wheat, yeast or corn).
                              This is a test for chemicals, especially
                              anti-staling agents which are present in
                              white bread retailed in the UK.

Day 32   peas (if frozen check no mint or sugar is
                          added)
                          grapefruit
                          pure honey

Day 33   cucumber

plaice
black pepper (condiment pepper)

Day 34 & 35   rye

Use Ryvita (the original rye crispbread). Take rye at every meal for two full days unless a reaction occurs earlier. If you should react to rye and you have already reacted to wheat, I do not think it is worth while testing oats or malt later, as reactions to these will by now be a foregone conclusion. It is wise to eat rye a little cautiously if a wheat allergy has already been detected. Rye and wheat are very closely related in the botanical tables and many people who are allergic to wheat will soon sensitize themselves to rye if they eat a lot of it. It is the most common cause of confusion and dismay on the last part of this elimination diet.

Day 36   instant coffee

Test Nescafé Gold Blend. This is another chemical test, predominantly for preserving chemicals. Caution — many cheap instant coffees contain corn.

asparagus
lemon

Day 37   olive oil
lentils
tinned carrots

Do not test tinned carrots if you are allergic to carrots! The object of this test is to test the phenolic resin lining of tins. These linings are present in many tins, and tinned carrots are selected as a convenient example. You should check that the tin contains no sugar if you are allergic to cane sugar, beet sugar, or glucose.

Day 38   monosodium glutamate

This is a flavour enhancer used in many tinned foods, sauces, gravies, etc. It can be obtained in pure white crystalline form in many supermarkets (especially

Chinese and delicatessens). A little of the powder should be sprinkled like salt over some meat or almost any other foodstuff you prefer.

prawns or shrimps
Brussels sprouts

Day 39 & 40   oats
Ideally take porridge oats at every meal for two days or until a reaction occurs.

Day 41   saccharin (Sweetex drops)
turkey
red/green peppers

Day 42   raisins (do not test if you are allergic to grapes)
mixed herbs
pineapple (if not tested already)

Day 43   cauliflower
chocolate
Chocolate contains wheat, corn, and sugar. Do not test if you are allergic to any of these items.

natural dates (if not tested already)

Day 44   malt
Test for one full day. Take two teaspoons of malt extract at every meal.

End of Stage IV assessment

If you have tried all the foods at each stage, you will have in effect assessed 80 foods, which account for 95 per cent of what most people eat. Fruits such as cherries, plums, peaches, raspberries, gooseberries, and blackcurrants are, of course, seasonal in their fresh form and have not been included in this elimination procedure, which has been devised to be used at any time of the year. These fruits should be tested when they become available in their normal season.

Complicated manufactured foods, such as jams, confectionery, sauces, cakes, biscuits, gravies, pizzas, and alcoholic beverages are mostly mixtures of items already tested, such as sugar, wheat, corn, yeast, soy, and egg. If you have this sort of allergy you will have problems with many manufactured foods unless you have neutralization therapy. These foods may also contain certain chemicals which have been tested, such as anti-staling agents, monosodium glutamate, and saccharin.

They can also contain various food dyes, for example, which have not yet been tested. Should you find yourself reacting to a multiple food containing items you know you are safe with, but also some tartrazine or other dyestuff, then it might be an idea to obtain some separate food dyes from a delicatessen and test them separately. It is possible to make up two drops of the dye with ten drops of water. Two or three drops of the diluted dye can then be placed under the tongue with a pipette and any reaction observed. In general, reactions to dyes are a rarity in arthritis. Lists of multiple foods containing corn, wheat, yeast, milk, eggs, and soy can be found at the end of this chapter. There is also a list of the common constituents of various alcoholic beverages in Chapter 4.

At the end of Stage IV you should, therefore, have what is perhaps best termed a 'compatible diet'. Most people will have found that, of the 80 items tested, 70 or more are satisfactory. On the fac e of it this sounds quite nice, but very frequently the ten foods that are implicated are the most difficult ones to avoid. For those people who have to eat out a lot in the course of their occupation, neutralization is virtually essential. For people who eat mostly at home, avoidance may be a practical consideration, particularly if they can find less commonly eaten foods to substitute for foods like wheat. Items such as buckwheat, buckwheat flour, sago, tapioca, and chick-pea flour can be useful in this context. There are, of course, many excellent foods not tested on the above 80-food test regime, but anyone who has been through that regime will now know how to go about food testing, and any of these items can now be tested and added to your repertoire. I include a list of such foods, largely to jog your memory.

114 Foods not included on elimination diet
Vegetables (27)

alfalfa	broad (fava)
artichokes	kidney
aubergines	butter (lima)
bamboo shoots	beansprouts
beans, various	celeriac
inc: aduki	chicory

garden cress
gherkins
kelp
okra
peas, various,
inc: black-eyed
    chick-peas (garbanzo)
    cream
    split
pumpkin
radishes
sago palm
salsify
squashes (various)
tapioca
watercress
yams

Fowl (7)
duck
goose
grouse
Guinea fowl
pheasant
pigeon
quail

Meats (3)
rabbit
hare
venison (deer)

Fruits (24)
apricots
blackberries
blueberries
cantaloupe
cherries
clementines
crab apples
cranberries
elderberries
gooseberries

kiwi fruit
limes
loganberries
mandarins
mangoes
nectarines
pomegranates
plums
prunes
raspberries
satsumas
strawberries
tangerines
ugli fruit

Nuts (10)
almonds
Brazil nuts
cashew nuts
chestnuts
filberts
hazelnuts
macadamia nuts
pecans
pistachios
walnuts

Grains (4)
barley
buckwheat
millet
wild rice

Salt and freshwater fish (24)
anchovies
brill
bream
carp
caviar
eel
haddock
hake
halibut

huss
monkfish
mullet
perch
salmon
sardines
sea bass
sea herring
sole
squid/octopus
swordfish
tunafish
turbot
whitebait
whiting

Shellfish (8)
cockles

crab
lobster
mussels
oysters
scallops
whelks
winkles

Miscellaneous (7)
herbal tea
green tea
China tea
goat's milk
sheep's milk
rhubarb
arrowroot

This list of 114 foods does not contain the enormous range of individual herbs and spices which is available. It also does not contain many occasionally available foods. Various exotic fish and tropical fruits, for example, are now beginning to appear in markets and restaurants as world-wide communication and affluence increase.

All these foods are individual biological entities. As such they may not be tolerated by sufferers with complex food allergy problems. In people who have a simple food allergy problem of three or four commonly-eaten foods, they are all likely to be tolerated well.

These foods can gradually be reintroduced into the diet at your leisure. Many people, especially those with very conservative eating habits, will probably eat hardly any of these items prior to a food allergy investigation. The general attitude of doctors in this field is, however, to encourage their patients to eat as wide a range of foods as possible. As allergy mostly seems to relate to the frequency of ingestion of specific foods, the less frequently any individual food is consumed the more likely you are to remain tolerant to it. To prevent the development of further food sensitivities, therefore, you should make a point of eating as wide a range of foods and varying them as much as possible (see Chapter 2).

Many people, when they first attend my clinic, tell me proudly that they eat very simply and never vary their diet. They consider it a virtue, but they are in fact wrong and it is probably the reason that they need to attend my clinic in the first place.

Cheeses

Cheeses present a distinct problem on elimination diets. Obviously if the cheese is manufactured partly from cow's milk and you are allergic to this it is likely (but not certain) that you will react to the cheese. Cheeses are complex mixtures of foods and, as their constituents are trade secrets, it is very difficult to obtain a list like, for example, the alcohol list on page 55. The *'Cheese Regulations'* obtainable from the Ministry of Agriculture Fisheries & Food is not a lot of help in this respect in that it just lists items that are permitted in certain cheeses. However, these possibilities are quite wide and the best solution really is to try out the cheeses individually after the main exclusion diet has finished. Cheeses commonly tried include Bel Paese, Brie, Camembert, Cheshire, Cottage cheese, Edam, Emmenthal, Gorgonzola, Gouda, Gruyere, Parmesan, Roquefort, Stilton and Swiss. Cheddar cheese has been evaluated on the original diet.

Alcohol

In Chapter 4, there is a list of alcoholic beverages related to their particular constituents. Again we are dealing with trade secrets, but the list is reasonably accurate for most brands of alcoholic beverages. If you are sensitive to yeast you will react adversely to all alcoholic beverages, though less probably to vodka and other spirits than to wine, as the spirits have been through a distillation process in which a lot of the yeast gets left behind. Neutralization therapy will usually allow individuals to drink alcoholic beverages containing one of their food allergens. However, as the food is absorbed so dramatically when it is part of an alcoholic beverage, it may give a slight reaction despite neutralization.

There now follow some helpful lists of foods containing wheat, corn, milk, yeast, and soy. Most of our patients opt for neutralization therapy after seeing these lists, but it is in fact possible to eat well avoiding all these manufactured items. It does, however, mean sticking to a whole food diet of simple meats, fowl, fish, fruit, vegetables, grains, nuts, etc.

Foods containing wheat

Breads
Biscuits
Cereal-derived sauces
Cheese spreads containing
  cereal products as fillers
Chocolate (all except bitter
chocolate)
Coffee substitutes
Commercial cakes
Crackers made from wheat
Commercial salad dressings
made with wheat flour
Canned and frozen foods
(some)
Flour
Gravies
Ice cream
Ice cream cones
Luncheon meats
Macaroni
Malt
Meat loaf
Meat or fish rissoles
Noodles
Pastas
Oatmeal (some)
Ovaltine
Pastries and pies
Puddings
Pancakes
Sausages
Soups thickened with wheat
flour
Any sauce or gravy thickened
with wheat flour
Spaghetti
Tortillas
Vermicelli
Waffles
Various alcoholic beverages
Most beers, whiskies and gins

Foods containing corn

Adhesives (envelopes, stamps,
  stickers)
Bacon (some)
Baking mixtures
Baking powders
Batters
Biscuits
Bleached wheat flour
Breads and pastries (some)
Carbonated beverages (most)
Cakes
Cheeses (some)
Chilli
Chocolate
Cornflakes
Cough syrups
Cream pies
Canned peas
Custards
Coated rice
Canned fruits (some)
Dates (sweetened)
Deep fat frying mixtures
Frozen fruits (some)
Fruit juices (some)
Gelatin desserts
Glucose products
Grape juice (some)
Gravies
Gum
Hams (some)
Ice cream
Icing sugar
Inhalants (bath and body
  powders)
Instant coffee (some)

Instant teas (some)
Jams
Jellies
Milk in paper cartons
Margarine
Peanut butter
Popcorn
Preserves
Puddings
Salad dressings
Sandwich spreads
Sauces
Sundaes
Sherbets
Starch (cornflour)
String beans – canned and
   frozen (some)
Soups
Soya milks (some)

Syrups
Sweeteners
Sweets
Tortillas
Vanilla
Vegetables – canned and
   frozen (some)
Vinegar (some)
Most tablets, capsules,
   lozenges, suppositories

Alcohol:
  Most beers
        whiskies
        gins
        sherries
        cheap wines
        (see alcohol list)

Foods containing milk or milk products

Au gratin foods (potatoes,
   beans)
Baking powder biscuits
Baker's bread
Boiled salad dressings
Bologna
Butter
Buttermilk
Butter sauces
Cakes
Candies
Cheese
Chocolate or cocoa drinks
Chowders
Cream
Creamed foods
Cream sauces
Curd
Custards
Doughnuts
Eggs, scrambled

Gravy
Hamburger buns
Junket
Ice cream
Mashed potatoes
Malted milk
Meat loaf
Milk (condensed, dried,
   evaporated, powdered)
Mixes for:
   biscuits
   cakes
   doughnuts
   muffins
   pancakes
   pie crust
   puddings
   waffles
Omelettes
Margarine
Quiche

Rarebits
Salad dressings
Sherbets
Soda Crackers
Souffles

Soups
Waffles
Whey
Yogurt

Foods containing yeast

1. Foods that contain yeast as an additive ingredient:
    Breads
    Biscuits
    Pastries
    Pretzels
    Hamburgers
    Hot dog rolls
    Cakes and cake mix
    Flour enriched with yeast vitamins
    Rolls and buns
    Milk fortified with vitamins from yeast
    Foods fried in bread crumbs

2. The following substances contain yeast or yeast-like substances because of their nature or the nature of their manufacture or preparation:
    Mushrooms, truffles, cheeses of all kinds, buttermilk, and cottage cheese.

    Various vinegars, such as apple, pear, grape, and distilled vinegar. These vinegars can also occur in mayonnaise, olives, pickles, sauerkraut, condiments, horseradish, French dressings, salad dressings, barbecue sauce, tomato sauce, chilli peppers, and mince pies.

    All alcoholic beverages – whiskies, gins, wines, brandy, rum, vodka, beer, etc.

    Malted products: cereals, sweets, chocolates, and milk drinks which have been malted.

    Citrus fruit juices, either frozen or canned. Almost all commercial citrus fruit juices contain yeast.

3. Many vitamin products are derived from yeast or have their sources from yeast.

Foods containing soya beans

1. Bakery goods
Soya bean flour containing only 1 per cent of oil is now used by some bakeries in their dough mixtures for breads, rolls, cakes, and pastries. This keeps them moist and saleable several days longer. The roasted nuts are used in place of peanuts.

2. Sauces
Oriental soya sauce   La Choy Sauce
Lea & Perrins Sauce   Heinz Worcestershire Sauce

3. Salad dressing
Many salad dressings and mayonnaises contain soya oil but only state on the label that they contain vegetable oil.

4. Meats
Pork sausage and luncheon meats may contain soya beans

5. Sweets
Soya flour is used in hard sweets. Lecithin is invariably derived from soya beans and is used in sweets to prevent drying out and to emulsify the fats.

6. Milk substitutes
Some bakers use soya milk instead of cows' milk.

7. Ice cream

8. Soups

9. Vegetables
Fresh soya sprouts are served as a vegetable, especially in Chinese dishes.

10. Soya nuts are roasted, salted, and used instead of peanuts.

11. Soya bean noodles, macaroni, and spaghetti.

12. Margarine and butter substitutes.

10 Neutralization and desensitization to foods

After identifying food sensitivity as being extremely important in most cases of arthritis, I became concerned that those of my patients who had multiple food sensitivities were finding it enormously difficult or impossible to avoid them completely. The problem is further complicated by the fact that the foods most frequently implicated are those which are the most difficult to avoid.

As can easily be imagined, sufferers with, for example, allergies to wheat, corn, milk and eggs would find it very difficult to attend a cocktail party, a wedding reception, a business dinner, or almost any other major social occasion. To attend such a function they would either appear to be an obsessional food faddist or alternatively be resigned to the inevitable joint pain which would occur a few hours after deviating from the diet. A quick perusal of the lists of foods containing corn, wheat, yeast, eggs, soy, cow's milk, etc. appearing in Chapter 9 will confirm these avoidance problems.

Allergists who have worked for years giving patients arbitrary and increasing doses of injected allergens for inhaled allergy problems have known that occasionally patients would report a startling improvement in their condition within an hour or so of receiving an allergy injection. This improvement would often last for nearly a week. Such patients would often return and ask for a futher injection (exactly the same as the last one). This rapid relief puzzled most allergists. It was considered by most to be a psychological quirk.

However, in 1957 Dr Carleton H. Lee of Kansas, Missouri, made the discovery which explained this curious phenomenon, and opened up the most amazing vistas for the control of allergic responses to foods, inhaled allergens, chemicals, and even hormones and viruses. Dr Lee's wife had severe asthma which he had discovered was related to the consumption of certain common foods. Unfortunately she reacted to a huge range of foods and could remain well only on two or three specific foods. Other foods would quickly bring on moderate or severe asthmatic attacks within a few hours.

Although food extract injection therapy had never before been found to have had any use, Dr Lee persisted in experimenting with injecting food extracts in the hope of helping his wife's problem. He eventually discovered to his delight that he could produce asthmatic symptoms with one carefully measured dose of food extract injected intradermally (between the layers of the skin). More importantly he found that another specific concentration would relieve this asthma within 10 minutes. This specific dose became known as the neutralizing dose. He then went on to observe that this specific dose, when given by a small subcutaneous injection (just under the skin), would protect his wife for the next two or three days should she eat that particular food. A cocktail of all the neutralizing doses of the foods to which she was sensitive, administered in a single injection about three times a week, would enable her to eat normally without any asthma.

Thus was born provocation neutralization testing and treatment. The word provocation refers to the production of symptoms with one dose of the injected allergen. The term neutralization relates to the relief of symptoms with another dose. Neutralization therapy is the treatment of the problem by low, tailor-made doses of the allergen, usually and most effectively administered by subcutaneous injection. Administration can also be effected with sublingual (under the tongue) drops, which is discussed in Chapter 13.

Soon Dr Lee discovered that he could utilize the same principles to 'neutralize' reactions to inhaled allergens, such as house dust, dust mites, moulds, animal furs, and summer pollens. It had been possible to treat such problems before with conventional incremental desensitization, but the success rate was low (often below 20 per cent) and the treatment took months or years to work. The relief with inhaled allergen neutralizing injections often starts within half an hour of the first neutralizing injection being administered and lasts for several days.

Safety

In 1986 in Great Britain desensitization treatment suddenly

made the headlines in the national press. The Committee on Safety in Medicines, a Government-appointed watchdog on the Pharmaceutical Industry, suddenly ruled that conventional incremental desensitization should be administered only by doctors working in units where there was adequate resuscitative equipment and the knowledge to use it. Furthermore, they ruled that patients were to remain in the units for an hour or so until it was quite certain that no very adverse response to the injection had occurred.

Up to the time of this ruling, most of the incremental desensitizing injections had been given rather casually in doctors' surgeries and often the patient had been allowed to go home immediately. Many GPs have not been well trained in how to deal with the adverse allergic reactions that these injections often initiated. As a result of this situation there had been, over the previous few years, a handful of patients who had died as a direct result of this type of treatment. Most of these patients were severe asthmatics who are in any case amongst the most difficult patients to treat in the whole field of allergic practice.

As a result of the 1986 ruling, incremental desensitization virtually stopped in the United Kingdom, except in a few allergy units in National Health Service hospitals. Although the safety of incremental desensitization was probably much higher than many still-used drugs, such as the anti-inflammatory drugs used by the million for treating arthritis, the benefit/risk ratio was low.

Risks with a specific treatment are often tolerated if the potential benefits of that treatment are high. The potential benefits, however, of incremental desensitization are very low. Only about 15 per cent of patients benefit from desensitization to allergens such as house dust, dust mite, and moulds. The success rate with desensitization to animal furs is even lower. Summer pollen desensitization is more successful, but because the season is limited, summer problems are usually less of a strain on patients than allergens which affect them all year round, such as house dust.

In contrast, with provocative neutralization therapy we observe almost total safety. There has not to my knowledge been a single fatality recorded anywhere in the world as a result of provocative neutralization therapy or testing. Currently there are only about 15 clinics using this method in the UK. There are, however, probably over 800 clinics in the USA using this technique. Provocative neutralization is used as the method of choice by members of the American Academy of Environmental

Medicine, the American Academy of Otolaryngolic Allergy, and the Pan American Allergy Society. The combined membership of these large societies exceeds 2,000 physicians and all these socieities run annual instructional courses for physicians interested in the technique.

In the UK, my clinic pioneered provocative neutralization testing in 1977, but many American clinics had been using it for years prior to this. Dr Carleton H. Lee made his initial observations in 1957 and treated many patients in the years after this. Dr Joseph Miller became interested in 1965 and had gained so much experience in it by 1972 that the published his book, *Food Allergy: Provocative Testing and Injection Therapy*. This became the 'bible' for many other American allergists who started treating patients in this manner soon after. In 1987 Lee published a further definitive book about his technique entitled, *Allergy Neutralization: The Lee Method*.

At least 10 million patients, at a conservative estimate, have received this form of treatment over a period of many years, without any fatalities. Most of these patients were in the USA or Canada, but many thousands were treated in the UK or Australia.

This safety factor is not surprising when one considers that the provocation neutralization method uses doses that are frequently several thousand times weaker than those used in incremental desensitization. Furthermore, the tailor-made doses employed for neutralization are ones which:

a) have a completely negative skin reaction
b) have an immediate positive health benefit.

In 1987 the Committee on Safety in Medicines acknowledged that their strictures concerning incremental desensitization did not apply to low-dose neutralization therapy, which they had not considered in their deliberations.

The technique

Food extracts are obtained from the usual allergy supply companies in the standard 1/10 or 1/20 prick test concentrations containing glycerine. The glycerine is added during the initial extraction process to stabilize the food extract so that it maintains its potency for many years. The dilutant that most clinics use nowadays is benzyl alcohol, as it has a very low incidence of allergy in itself. The benzyl alcohol is prepared in intravenous-quality normal saline and, using this dilutant, nine separate dilutions, a serial 1/5 dilution, are prepared. Thus dilutions of 1/5, 1/25, 1/125, 1/625 and so on are prepared for testing. The test consists of giving intradermal injections of varying concentrations of the foods known or suspected to be causing the patient's problems. Testing usually begins on the 1/25 strength and if a positive reaction is obtained the doctor proceeds at 10-minute intervals to weaker strengths.

In assessing wheals there are various criteria. When 1/20 cc of a food extract is injected intradermally it will produce a wheal which at the time of injection is hard, raised, blanched and has well-demarcated edges. After 10 minutes a positive wheal will usually have retained most of these features and will have grown at least 2mm in diameter. Negative wheals lose these characteristics and grow less than 2mm.

If the initial injection results in a positive wheal, with or without symptoms, the physician moves to a consecutively weaker strength until the first negative wheal is found. This is the neutralizing dose and also the treatment concentration, unless symptoms induced by the stronger strength have not entirely cleared, in which case a move to the next weaker solution will normally clear them. In over 80 per cent of cases the first negative wheal is the neutralizing dose. If a weaker dose than the neutralizing dose is administered, then symptoms will usually recur. This is called under-dosage and the symptoms can be removed by going back to the stronger dose which is obviously the neutralizing level. Thus, in someone suffering from arthritis, joint pains can be induced by too strong or too weak a dose and can be removed by the neutralizing dose. People find it amazing that their joint pains and swelling can be turned on and off within a few minutes. They often find the changes so impressive that they wish medical sceptics could observe the changes they were experiencing in their own bodies.

In April 1985 there was a BBC TV *Horizon* broadcast on the topic of food allergy, watched by over 11 million people. The programme opened with a video recording of an American physician with severe arthritis, who had been treated by Dr Marshall Mandell, who practises in New England. It showed a short sequence of this severely arthritic doctor walking with obvious great pain and difficulty. Several minutes later, after a neutralizing injection had been given, this same doctor was able to walk easily and with virtually no pain. Later in the same

programme I showed a female patient with rheumatoid arthritis
having pain induced in her hands with a 1/25 extract of wheat,
followed by total relief a few minutes later after the injection of a
1/625 extract of wheat. The programme evoked a great deal of
interest on the part of the general public and in the newspapers,
but unhappily very little from the medical profession, who
appear to lack curiosity about these interesting phenomena.

These techniques do after all lend themselves to fairly simple
scientific evaluation. The patient has no way of knowing
whether a testing nurse or physician is using an active extract or
a dummy, 'placebo' injection, for example normal saline. I have
frequently demonstrated to physicians visiting my clinic that
patients can identify from their clinical responses whether they
are being injected with one of their known allergens or a
placebo. These physicians are usually highly impressed and
often go off to do the same work themselves. However, until the
higher echelons of the medical profession, the teaching hospital
professors and so forth become interested, dissemination of this
knowledge is going to be painfully slow and in the meantime
millions of patients with severe joint problems are going to
continue to suffer.

Clinical trials have, however, been performed on neutraliztion
therapy already and these have been published in various
journals. They are detailed in Chapter 13.

How neutralization therapy works

Currently we know a certain amount about the immunologic
process that is involved in the neutralization phenomenon. The
fine details, however, are not as yet fully understood and I think
it may well be many years before they are. This problem,
however, applies to most medical treatments currently available.

- We do not know how painkillers work.
- We do not know how sleeping tablets work.
- We do not know how anti-inflammatory drugs work in
  relieving pain and swelling in arthritis.
- We do not know how gold injections work in rheumatoid
  arthritis.
- We do not know how conventional incremental
  desensitization works (or does not work!).

I could go on for a long time in this vein. Most drug treatment has been discovered by chance in a very empirical fashion. New drugs are usually discovered by trying out whole ranges of new synthetic chemicals on animals such as guinea pigs and rats. Those which appear to have the more beneficial effects are then tried on 'higher' animals, such as cats. After animal experimentation the more promising-looking drugs are then tried on human volunteers. The whole process is therefore based much more on trial and error than on any great understanding of the basic mechanism of the disease process that is being considered.

In order to give some idea as to how neutralization works, it is necessary to enter into the whole world of immunology. In immunology we have on one hand allergenic molecules, but these molecules have to react on an organ to produce a reaction. The organ that produces a reaction is called a stress organ. In the case of arthritis the stress organ is the joint or joints, or perhaps more precisely the synovial membrane lining the joints.

Allergenic molecules of food or inhalants cause reaction in stress organs through two types of cell, mast cells and basophils. These cells release histamine granules and other potentially harmful chemicals. Mast cells were called such because under the microscope they look like bags of mast (a container of nuts, seeds and acorns). Mast cells are found on the outer surface of capillary blood vessels just under the skin or around the capillaries in the mucous membranes of the respiratory or digestive tracts. Mast cells cling to the capillaries like a great swarm of bees clinging to the branches of a tree.

Basophils in contrast normally reside in the bloodstream itself and circulate around the whole body. When necessary basophils have the ability to enter tissues through breaks in the capillary blood vessels. They can then release their granules and other chemicals to help the effects of their sister cell, the mast cell. The chemicals, especially histamine, released by these two cells cause the allergic reaction. Other chemicals that they release, called prostaglandins and leucotrienes, can be quite harmful and they can in turn stimulate other types of cell to arrive at the reaction site and release further potentially harmful chemicals to fight antigens that are more difficult to overcome. This mechanism increases the response to the antigen, but these extra chemicals may well cause destruction of normal tissue. Thus the reaction changes from a purely allergic response to an inflammation (arthritis).

The skin is composed of two layers, the epidermis (outer layer)

Figure 3   Composition of the skin

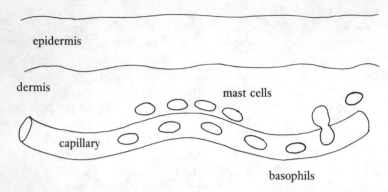

epidermis

dermis   mast cells

capillary

basophils

and dermis (inner layer). Mast cells are attrached to the outer surface of the capillaries. Basophils normally circulate in the capillaries, but can leave them when needed.

The chemical mediators released from mast cells and basophils can occur not only as a reaction to allergenic molecules, but also as a reaction to virus infections, excessive cold, and certain hormonal changes.

When an intradermal injection is administered, it stimulates the vast network of highly reactive immunologic cells situated in the skin. Allergens injected into the epidermis or superficial layer of the skin can make the mast cells surrounding the capillaries sting them like a bee. The venom from this sting (chemical mediators) forces the local capillaries, which are only one cell thick, to contract and become slightly separated from each other, opening up tiny crevices between them.

The gaps so caused allow a two-way flow from the tissues into the capillaries and from the capillaries into the bloodstream. Injected antigen and some chemical mediators enter the bloodstream, and watery blood serum containing basophils and chemicals leaks out into the tissues while the reaction is occurring.

This increased flow between the capillaries and the surrounding tissue is critical to all allergic or inflammatory reactions. The body can excrete harmful allergens quickly from the bloodstream and deposit them in the tissues where they will usually be less of a problem, and it can send protective substances, such as antibodies, quickly out of the bloodstream through these capillary gaps.

Neutralization occurs when a homoeostatic balance is achie-

Figure 4 Two-way flow between capillaries and antigen wheals, and between capillaries and tissues

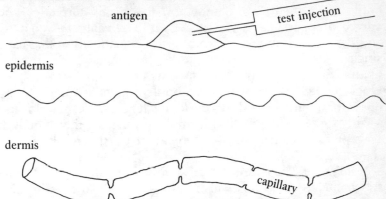

ved in this two-way process. Immunologists are learning that these homoeostatic controlling mechanisms are incredibly complex and numerous. There are many reaction stimulating or suppressing factors.

The immune system is like a million huge armies which have many weapons and strategies co-ordinated to oppose similarly huge armies of allergens, bacteria, viruses, fungi, yeasts, and toxins.

The homoeostatic restoring dose of the offending substance that is given in neutralization therapy drives the system back towards a normal balance. It usually levels out the tilted balance within a few minutes and turns off the release or harmful effects of histamine and the other chemical mediators much more effectively and quickly than any other technique known to mankind.

Administration of neutralization

After the neutralizing levels for the major food allergens have been determined, they are either administered to the patient by sublingual drops or by subcutaneous injections, which are usually self-administered. Sublingual drops are so called because they are placed beneath the tongue. The area under the human tongue is an area of high absorbability. Inspection of the area under the tongue will reveal large veins which are called the sublingual veins, and absorption is effective in this area. This is, of course, the reason why patients who are taking nitroglycerine tablets to treat angina place these tablets under their tongue to obtain the most rapid response. Sublingual desensitizing drops are therefore placed under the tongue using a special dropper bottle and patients are taught how to do this correctly. The curved dropper bottles produce a carefully calibrated quantity and the solution in the dropper bottles is made up so that each single drop delivered from the pipette contains the precise neutralizing dose of the food to which the patient is sensitive. One drop delivered from such a bottle can contain neutralizing doses for a number of different food allergens. Technicians use a fairly simple mathematical formula to calculate the amount of reagent each patient needs, dependent on the results of the skin-testing.

Sublingual drops are effective for about five hours, while subcutaneous injections will be effective for two days in most patients. The injections are normally made up in 0.5cc dosage and the amount of food allergens in these is of course caluclated appropriately. Of the two methods my preference is for the subcutaneous injections, although I do use both. Nowadays modern insulin syringes are disposable, have a very fine built-in needle, are extremely easy to use and, most important of all, very rarely hurt when you inject yourself. Most people who try both methods of administering their neutralizing doses prefer the injection because it is more effective, and the fact that it is only required every two days makes it very convenient.

These desensitizing drops or injections fulfil two purposes. The first is that, within a day or so, they enable you to eat the food to which you are sensitive, without adverse effect. Secondly, if the desensitization has been administered for a couple of years or so, patients become desensitized to the food and find they can eat it without recourse to drops or injections.

Diagnosis using skin-testing

An extension of this technique is to use it for diagnosis. Clearly, if positive wheal reactions and symptoms can be obtained in the course of desensitization, there is no need to go through an elimination dietary procedure. Furthermore, whereas an elimination dietary procedure can take five or six weeks, during which time you have to avoid major social occasions, a comprehensive skin-testing programme can be completed in about four days of intensive testing. A workable procedure in these circumstances is to scan about 34 major foods in intradermal provocation skin tests. The reaction to all 34 foods is tested, and neutralizing doses are obtained for all those items to which there is a positive reaction. The testing procedure on average takes about seven 2½–hour test sessions to complete. At the end of the testing programme, you are allowed to eat only those foods tested and take injections or drops to cover all those items to which sensitivity has been found.

The advantages of this approach are considerable.

- The testing programme is completed in a few days.
- You do not have to assess your own response.
- You do not have to abandon any drugs you are taking which can be either hazardous or extremely unpleasant.
- If you live a long way from the clinic, this test procedure saves a whole series of long journeys at various stages of the elimination diet.
- If you have multiple food allergies, these tests will be inevitable anyway, even after the elimination diet, because you will need to be desensitized to a large number of foods.
- In most cases the treatment programme is very successful.

The disadvantages of this treatment, as opposed to the elimination diet followed by desensitization to specifically identified food allergens, are:

- The skin-test technique picks up adapted food allergies as well as non-adapted allergies (see Chapter 2). Hence the number of foods to which someone reacts often appears more complicated than it really is, and a degree of over-treatment is almost inevitably present using this technique.
- You do not know that you are going to become completely well until after the treatment is completed, whereas after the first stage of the elimination diet most people can discover for themselves that, once removed from their major food allergies, they feel much better.
- Going through an elimination diet probably gives you a better idea than skin-testing as to which food allergens cause severe reactions and which mild, and also you may learn to associate certain symptoms with certain foods.
- The elimination diet is an educative programme, whereas skin-testing is far less so in itself. Consequently, at the end of a skin-testing programme, you must learn to use only those items which have been tested. This involves some education

into how multiple foods are made up and what they contain. For example, at the end of the testing programme, it is probable that wholemeal bread will be permitted in the diet, but not white bread because the chemicals (bleaching agents, anti-staling agents, etc.) added to this have not been assessed. At the end of such a programme you can sabotage all the careful work that has been done up to that point by, for example, eating white bread. If you are sensitive to the chemicals in white bread and are not covered for them by desensitizing drops or injections, this may in itself be enough to cause symptoms to recur.

After remaining on the foods tested for a few weeks and presumably being free of symptoms, you can then extend your repertoire of foods by bringing back into your diet one single food item at a time and testing it.

Disadvantages of neutralization therapy

By far the biggest problem with neutralization therapy is the fact that after several weeks or months of this treatment the neutralizing levels can change. Often the specific reason for this change is inexplicable, but in many cases it appears to be a feature of the progressive desensitization that is occurring as treatment continues to be administered. What normally happens is that someone who has experienced enormous or total relief of arthritis suddenly notices that joint pains are beginning to recur without any obvious change in the diet. In these circumstances retesting is necessary. Another possible reason for a change in neutralization levels is the occurrence of a severe attack of flu or a similar viral illness. Most frequently the retesting reveals that the neutralizing levels have become stronger. In other words, as individuals become progressively desensitized, they need a stronger dose to neutralize the symptoms. It is furthermore possible that several months later the neutralization levels will again change to an even stronger level, at which point the levels usually remain very stable. Certainly instability of neutralizing levels almost inevitably decreases with time.

The main disadvantage with changing neutralizing levels of course concerns the inevitable cost to the patient of retesting and, where necessary, taking time off work for this to be done. If only a few foods or inhalants are involved this is a minor problem, but it can be quite a big problem if multiple allergies are being dealt with. However, the ongoing cost of the neutralizing injections compares extremely favourably with the cost of anti-inflammatory drugs or Penicillamine taken over the same period of time.

The other problem with neutralization therapy is that we see some people who cannot be neutralized to a specific food. They may find that the technique works for nine foods, but does not work for the tenth. If any food is going to be a problem it is usually wheat and this is thought to be because wheat is quite complex allergically. If, however, the patient can be desensitized to rye (which is usually the case) it provides a reasonably good alternative.

Considering the enormous benefits of this technique, these disadvantages are quite small. There is, with the possible exception of a technique pioneered by Dr Len McEwen called enzyme potentiated desensitization, no other technique which enables allergy sufferers to eat foods to which they are sensitive. Enzyme potentiated desensitization has only a few active advocates and has, at the time of writing, been evaluated by only one major formal clinical trial. Provocative neutralization therapy has, however, been subjected to many trials which have established its effectiveness and it is currently used by several hundred physicians in their daily practice.

11 Neutralization to inhalants and chemicals

The chemical problem has been described and discussed in Chapter 3 and the inhalant problem in Chapter 5. The basic concept of neutralization for inhalants and chemicals is identical to that for foods, as described in the last chapter. The main difference, however, is that for inhaled allergens such as dust and dust mite the testing usually starts at a weaker strength. When testing food sensitivity the initial test dose is usually the No. 2 or 1/25 strength made from the concentrate obtained from the allergy supply company. For inhalant sensitivity is is normal to start two strengths lower, on the No. 4 strength or 1/625 strength.

The reasons for this are that some supersensitive people may react quite severely to a strong strength of an inhalant allergen, and the common neutralizing concentrations for inhalants are the 5, 6 and 7 levels. Obviously one wishes to get to the neutralizing level as quickly as possible for each item. The common neutralizing levels for food allergy are the 2, 3 and 4 levels. It is, I believe, because of this single fact that food allergy has been neglected for so long. Skin prick tests, for a long time the single arbiter of whether someone was allergic to something or not, are equivalent to giving a No. 4 (1/625) strength intradermally. In other words, all those who are prick-test positive will respond to a No. 4 level of the same item when administered intradermally, be it food or an inhalant. Because most food sensitivities neutralize on the 2, 3 or 4 levels, most foods tested by prick test are negative, even when genuine allergy is present. Most inhalants neutralize on the No. 5, 6 or 7 levels, so most inhalant prick tests show positivity when an inhalant sensitivity is present. There are, however, a substantial minority of patients with genuine inhalant allergy who neutralize on the 3 or 4 levels and these have in the past been missed by ordinary prick tests.

The logistics of sorting out inhaled allergy, therefore, fall into two categories:

1. sorting out which air-borne allergens are likely to be affecting the sufferer
2. obtaining the right neutralizing levels to each of these allergens.

Usually house dust and dust mite do not prove much of a problem but we have found it worthwhile to test both types of house dust mite, that is *D. pteronyssinus* and *D. farinae*. Testing individual animals, feathers, and wool is also fairly straightforward.

Mould sensitivity

A more difficult problem is mould sensitivity. There are over 20 separate moulds commonly floating in the atmosphere in the UK, and testing these all individually is both very time-consuming and expensive. Because of this the allergy supply companies also supply various mould mixtures, usually called something like Mould Mix A, B and C. Each of these mould mixtures contain about 8 separate moulds, and when testing with these mixtures a positive reaction presumably indicates a reaction to whichever mould in that mixture is giving the most trouble. Frequently neutralization with the mould mixtures is very effective, but sometimes it is quite disappointing. Presumably in some patients this is due to the fact that there may be significant reactions to two or more moulds in that particular mixture, all of which may have distinctly different neutralizing levels. The mould mixture cannot therefore be adequately neutralizing several different moulds at the same time.

This problem may be solved in some people by quickly prick-testing all the moulds and then neutralizing the patients to what appear to be the most significant reactors. Some sufferers have exposed mould culture plates in their homes to identify which particular mould seems to be the most prevalent in their environment. We have then tested them with these specific moulds.

Neutralization to chemicals in arthritis tends to have only marginal benefit, as the main problems in arthritis are the more constant exposures, such as gas, oil, and formaldehyde. Neutralizing constant chemical exposures is only very partially successful and avoidance by modification of the house is always the treatment of choice. Furthermore, neutralization treatment is given by sublingual drops to avoid the need for individuals to inject themselves with chemicals. Sublingual drops are effective for only four or five hours and they therefore need to be taken at regular intervals throughout the day if contact with the exposure is constant. Where I find neutralizing drops of gas extract to be most useful in day-to-day practice is with patients who have removed gas utilities from the interior of their own home but need protection when they visit their friends who still have gas utilities.

Occasionally encountered inhaled chemicals seem not to be a great problem with most arthritis sufferers, but there is the occasional exception. Sublingual neutralizing drops of petrol, diesel, cigarette smoke, perfumes, etc. are quite useful in these circumstances and are only taken when sufferers are exposed to their particular allergen.

It should be pointed out that chemical neutralizing drops give only temporary protection from symptoms and do not appear to eventually desensitize as we find with food and other inhalant allergies. Accordingly in the USA they are referred to as 'cheater drops' as all they do is temporarily cheat the symptoms.

What may lead to a permanent resolution of the chemical sensitivity problem is treatment for intestinal candidiasis. Chapter 6 of this book deals with this subject in some depth and, as stated in that chapter, it appears that many cases of chemical sensitivity are actually caused by the Candida problem. In the view of Dr Orion Truss, the now famous discoverer of the Candida problem, chemical sensitivity is almost always secondary to candidiasis. As he rightly says, many patients appear to lose their chemical sensitivity after aggressive treatment for their Candida problem.

It does appear, however, that most sufferers, especially those with sensitivity to constantly-contacted items such as natural gas, need a major rest from their exposure to enable their system to re-establish equilibrium.

Gas

The most common problem by far is gas, and by that I mean household gas nowadays derived from the North Sea. A classic case of gas sensitivity was the second case described in Chapter 1. As in this particular case the diagnosis is established in several steps.

step 1:   a history of improvement when away from chemical exposure or worsening when in contact arouses suspicion

step 2:   intradermal skin testing with synthetic ethanol and/or natural gas extract

step 3:   if step 2 is positive, we still do not know if the gas sensitivity contributes 5 per cent of the problem, 30 per cent or 80 per cent. Temporarily turning off all the gas utilities in the house combined with ventilating the house usually answers this question. If there is substantial improvement which then disappears on re-establishing the gas utilities, the diagnosis is then obvious to all. If there still remains any doubt, the procedure can be repeated by further turning off the gas, observing the response and then turning it on again.

Once the importance of gas is established, the first thing to do is to replace the gas cooker with an electric one. Any gas fires should be sealed off and replaced with electric ones. Gas central heating boilers should be moved from the kitchen, utility room or under the stairs to an outhouse. Obviously this would be impossible in a fifth-floor flat. Moving the gas boiler into an outhouse is an expensive business and it is not undertaken unless the value of this procedure has been proven as described.

Building an outhouse can cost £300-400 in Britain, and the plumbing needed to re-site the boiler can cost another £300-400 quite easily. Luckily when we moved to our current clinic the gas boiler could be moved to a redundant exterior toilet and the procedure cost us only £250 in toto.

Room-sealed boilers are becoming much more common in the UK, and some sufferers seem able to live with these without problems. I have been instrumental in several hundred gas boilers being resited in the UK. Dr Theron Randolph in the USA tells me that with his longer experience in the field he has caused several 'thousand American 'furnaces' to be moved. I have never had a patient regret the procedure.

Other constantly inhaled chemicals such as formaldehyde and the gas given off by soft plastic (phenol) are less common problems than gas. Soft plastics, if identified as a problem, are reasonably easy to remove from the house, but formaldehyde can be a major problem. In some houses the cavity walls are insulated with urea formaldehyde resin, and formaldehyde may heavily impregnated in the plaster boards, etc. There is also a lot of formaldehyde in many caravans. In the rare case when formaldehyde is identified as a major problem, moving house may be the only option, although this is only contemplated after steps similar to those described for confirming the gas problem have been completed.

12   Clinical trials of allergy and rheumatoid arthritis

Much of the evidence related in other parts of this book is of specific case histories and this type of evidence has become very suspect in the eyes of many doctors, as spontaneous remissions do occur in even quite severe illness. Case histories are, however, more scientifically valuable in this particular area of medicine as the 'remission' can usually be smartly reversed by re-eating the offending foods, if necessary in a double-blind fashion.

Nevertheless, physicians who have not realized the significance of this will continue to refer to case history studies as anecdotal. This word is defined in the *Concise Oxford Dictionary* as 'a narrative of an amusing or interesting incident'. This definition accurately reflects the derisory view of specific case histories in medical practice, as opposed to legal practice where the opposite view prevails.

Formal clinical trials are therefore necessary to establish the validity of this subject, although there is some difficulty in constructing them as the contributory factors vary so much from patient to patient.

I will detail the work done in this subject in chronological order. All the clinical trials performed related to rheumatoid arthritis. There are, as far as I know, no major organized trials verifying this approach in relation to osteoarthritis, ankylosing spondylitis, etc. Lay readers may find that some of the information in this chapter is difficult to understand without medical training. Clinical trials are complex affairs and with the best will in the world it is impossible to explain them simply. I want to include this chapter, however, especially for physicians.

As described in Chapter 2, various physicians in the early part of this century, such as Talbot in 1917 and Cooke in 1918, reported many cases of arthritis related to food sensitivitiy. Vaughan in 1943 reported 27 cases of recurrent or chronic arthritic symptoms, 13 of which he classified as rheumatoid arthritis due to food allergy. These findings were duplicated by Crisp in 1946 and Zussman in 1966. The famous allergist, Dr Albert Rowe, devoted a whole chapter to arthritis in his book *Food Allergy*, originally published in 1931 with further editions appearing up to 1972. In 1949 Dr Michael Zeller had a paper published in the *Annals of Allergy* entitled 'Rheumatoid Arthritis: Food Allergy as a Factor', an in-depth study of four patients whose rheumatoid arthritis had been shown to be apparently related to food sensitivity. Dr Zeller detailed his observations that symptoms of arthritis could frequently be relieved by appropriate food exclusion diets. He strongly emphasized his view that the subsequent reproduction of arthritic symptoms on reingestion of certain foods established the cause of that patient's rheumatoid arthritis. Repeated reintroduction of identified food allergens with a minimum of five-day intervals could be shown to repeatedly reproduce the arthritic responses on each occasion.

In Britain, the first serious work published on this subject was reported in the journal *Clinical Allergy* (1980, Vol. 10, page 463). The paper was authored by Dr Len McEwen who then worked in the Department of Allergy at St Mary's Hospital Paddington, and Dr Tony Hicklin of Redhill General Hospital. Dr McEwen in particular has continued to pioneer this approach with arthritis ever since. In their paper they stated that 22 patients with rheumatoid arthritis (15 seropositive) were asked to follow allergen-exclusion diets; 20 noticed an improvement in their symptoms, and 19 said that certain foods would repeatedly exacerbate symptoms of arthritis.

Food sensitivities reported were: grain 14, milk 4, pips and nuts 8, beef 4, cheese 7, egg 5, and one each of chicken, fish, potato, onion and liver — a mean of 2.5 unrelated food sensitivities per patient. With correct exclusion dieting the greatest delay before improvement noticed was 18 days — a mean of 10 days. There was great variation in the delay of reactions to dietary provocation. The shortest interval observed was two hours and the longest two weeks. Since sensitivity to all grain products was common in this series and because potato should be excluded from the initial diagnostic diet, sago was used as the main source of carbohydrate. The new exclusion diets are not excessively monotonous, but appear more efficient than previous alternatives for the investigation of food allergy.

In June 1981 the *British Medical Journal* (Vol. 282, page 2027) reported an in-depth case study from the Department of Rheumatology at Hammersmith Hospital, which is probably the most prestigious department of rheumatology in the world. The authors were Dr Graham Hughes, the Consultant at the Unit, and his Senior Registrar, Dr A.L. Parke.

The patient studied was a 38-year-old mother of three children who had an 11-year history of progressive, erosive, seronegative rheumatoid arthritis. Treatment with salicylates, non-steroidal anti-inflammatory drugs, Gold, Penicillamine and Prednisolone had all been dismal failures. She had severe joint pain and swelling affecting almost all her joints. Amongst other findings were very weak grip strengths, a high Ritchie index of arthritic activity and a high sedimentation rate of 110mm in the first hour.

It had been noted that the patient had a passion for cheese, consuming up to 1lb (450g) a day of this food. At the suggestion of the hospital she omitted cheese, milk and butter totally from her diet. Three weeks after she had omitted these foods she felt much improved and eventually all her symptoms abated. All the objective clinical tests returned to normal. The sedimentation rate dropped considerably and the circulating immune complexes in her serum, which had been high, disappeared. The improvement continued, except when she inadvertently ate dairy products, after which occasions the symptoms would recur within 12 hours.

At the suggestion of the Hammersmith Hospital the patient was admitted for specific challenge tests to prove the relationship of her arthritis to the milk products. In the first three days after admission she consumed 3lb of cheese and 7 pints (4 litres) of milk. The whole range of clinical and immunological measurements were performed before the challenge, 12 hours after the challenge and daily therafter.

Within 24 hours there was a pronounced deterioration of the patient's arthritis, with an increase in Ritchie index and morning stiffness and decreases in grip strength. The ring size of several fingers also increased, the largest increase being a change of 5mm. Laboratory measurements changed with the development of a leucocytosis and changes in concentration of circulating immune complexes. Results of RAST tests for IgE antibodies to milk and cheese proteins were negative before the challenge, but became positive during the challenge. The clearance of heat-damaged red cells was normal before the food challenge but

became considerably prolonged when tested two days and 14
days after the start of the challenge. All tests reverted to normal
six weeks after the challenge period. It is more than a little
difficult to dispute that milk products were the cause of this
lady's problems.

Two months after this paper appeared in the *British Medical
Journal*, Dr R. Williams wrote to the same journal describing the
case history of a patient whom he had referred to me some
couple of years before. The patient it referred to was a charming
woman who was the Mother Superior of a Convent. Dr
Williams has given me permission to reproduce his letter in full.

Rheumatoid arthritis and food: a case study
'SIR, — The paper by Drs A.L. Parke and G.R.V. Hughes (20
June, p. 2027) entitled 'Rheumatoid arthritis and food: a case
study', printed under the general heading 'For Debate', seems
to have produced no correspondence at all, which I find
surprising. I suspect that the doctors who work in the field of
food allergies are more anxious at present to get on with their
work and establish their ground scientifically than to stir up a
hornets' nest of correspondence, and I for one do not blame
them. But many GPs already know of equally dramatic cases, in
both rheumatoid arthritis and osteoarthritis.

The most impressive patient in my own experience had had
active rheumatoid arthritis for 25 years, was taking azathioprine
and soluble aspirins (Disprin), had already had a plasma
exchange and was slowly but steadily going downhill. She also
had proved pulmonary involvement, which meant an increased
anaesthetic risk from the splenectomy which had been contemplated. Her most important food allergen proved to be corn,
which, of course, as maize starch, was the packing in her
azathioprine and Disprin tablets. There was no question of
stopping her azathioprine or Disprin at that stage and it was
therefore necessary to counter any possible allergic effect of the
corn in her tablets by a simple method which there is not space
to go into here. Her improvement after one week on an
exclusion diet was so dramatic that the experiment seemed
worth pursuing, but after six weeks her arthritis flared badly and
it seemed that, sadly, the placebo effect of a new approach had
worn off. It transpired, however, that during that week cornflour
thickening had been added to her gravy against instructions and
without her knowledge and as soon as this was stopped her
joints resumed their improvement. Her erythrocyte sedimenta-

tion rate fell steadily from 75 to 31 in one hour and she began to put on weight. She is now off all tablets and feeling and looking better than she has done for over 20 years. I saw her five weeks ago and can confirm this. She attends hospital at three-month intervals instead of weekly and, as the staff freely admit, she goes there in their interest, not hers. Her chest X-ray appearances have become clear and her lung function has returned, she believes, to normal.

Of course this case is anecdotal, like that reported by Drs Parke and Hughes, in which the food allergen proved to be dairy produce. But both happened. The investigation required is simple, safe, and non-invasive, and it costs virtually nothing. All that is required is a co-operative patient with the will to persevere, careful instruction sheets, which already exist, and a doctor to monitor the experiment. One knows within a week, or at the most 10 days, whether the thing is worth pursuing. It will not be clear at that stage what the food allergen is, but there will be strong indications whether one does or does not exist and the patient will be in no doubt at all.

No one would be foolish enough to claim that every case of rheumatoid arthritis is associated with a food allergy, but if only one in 20 is — and I suspect that it is considerably more — I question whether we have the right to withhold such a simple, safe, brief, and non-invasive investigation in a disease of such appalling chronicity.'

Perhaps the most all-embracing trial yet performed was carried out in three major environmental control units in the USA. These units were the Comprehensive Environmental Control Centre in Chicago which was originally set up by Dr Theron Randolph, the Dallas Environmental Centre headed by Dr William J Rea, and the South Eastern Rheumatology and Allergy Centre, Chadbourn, North Carolina, headed by Dr Murray Carroll.

The trial unfortunately was not published in a major international journal, probably because its findings were so controversial. Instead it was published in the *Journal of Clinical Ecology* which is mostly read by allergists and physicians already interested in this particular subject. Physicians wishing to study all the details of this trial can obtain the magazine from Clinical Ecology Publications, 109 West Olive Street, Fort Collins, CO 80524, USA. The trial was published in two parts. The first part, entitled 'Fasting and Rheumatoid Arthritis', was published in Vol. II, No. 3, pp. 137-45. The second part, entitled 'Food Challenge Effects on Rheumatoid Arthritis Patients', was published in Vol. II, No. 4, pp. 181-9. The summary of the first part of this trial stated that 43 patients with definite or classical rheumatoid arthritis from three hospital centres underwent a water fast lasting 6.6 days on average under controlled environmental conditions. No major medical complications were noted. Seven parameters of arthritic activity (Tenderness Articular Indices, Swelling Articular Indices, Grip Strength, Dolorimeter Pain Index, Arthrocircameter, PIP Joint Circumference, Functional Activity Index Questionnaire, and ESR significantly improved (P < 0.001) during the fast).

These patients had all been admitted to environmental control units as described in Chapter 3. The majority of patients had had treatment with non-steroidal anti-inflammatory drugs, Gold or steroids prior to their admission. Many had experienced adverse drug reactions, especially to gold salts. All medications were immediately discontinued except for a maintenance dose of about 5mg of Prednisolone in three of the 43 patients. Walking around the wards was encouraged, to counter any suggestion that bed rest was responsible for the improvement. Before and during the water fast daily sequential measurements were taken to quantify grip strength, joint tenderness, joint swelling and other factors.

The table opposite gives the findings obtained and speaks for itself.

Of particular interest to me was the mean decline in the sedimentation rate noted during this fast. The decline was 13mm in the first hour, which is a much higher figure than is normally obtained within a few days of any drug therapy. At the end of the fast, 80.6 per cent of the patients had fair to excellent responses. Fair refers to a percentage improvement of 25-50 per cent; good refers to improvements of 50-75 per cent; and excellent refers to improvements greater than 75 per cent. There were poor responses in 19.4 per cent of patients, who had more advanced and long-standing problems accompanied by considerable joint destruction. Although this does not appear in the actual published trial, I gather that the poor responders were mostly patients who had had prolonged steroid treatment, which is definitely a very adverse factor when assessing the outlook for patients undergoing this form of treatment.

In the second part of this trial, 27 patients from the initial fasting study were then subjected to single sequential primary

Changes in 7 arthritic parameters measured before and after fasting in rheumatoid arthritis patients

Measurement	Measurement Change during Fasting			
	No.	Improved	No Change	Worse
Grip Strength** (mm Hg)	39	34	1	4
Dolorimeter** pain index	39	35	2	2
Swelling index**	43	41	1	1
Pain index**	43	41	2	0
Sedimentation rate* westergren (mm/hr)	33	28	1	4
Functional Activity* index	32	21	6	5
Arthrocircameter* PIP jt swelling (mm)	35	27	3	5

** Three hospital centres
* Two hospital centres

organic food challenges. Three meals a day were given to these patients. A single new food was tried at each meal unless the patient was already reacting to an earlier food. At the end of the organic food challenge period, patients were re-challenged with commercial foods which were previously non-reactive in their organic form. These commercial foods contained food additives, such as artificial colourings, flavour enhancers, antioxidants, and traces of pesticides.

In the course of the food challenges all symptoms were recorded, including of course joint symptoms. These symptoms were quantified by the nursing staff who also performed the whole range of standard rheumatologic measurements after each meal. The mean values taken after negative challenges were considered to be the baseline for each patient, when compared to the measurements made after the reactive foods. It should be noted that the non-reactive food baseline was, for most patients, completely asymptomatic.

A total of 735 organic food challenges were performed on the 27 patients. An average of 27.2 foods were tested per patient, of which 19 foods were found to be non-reactive, 5.7 foods mildly to moderately reactive, and 3.1 foods to be severely reactive. A total of 512 out of the 735 food challenges showed no reaction at all.

Superimposed on this control baseline most rheumatoid patients in this trial responded to specific foods with acute inflammatory reactions. The objective parameters measured after these specific reactions showed statistically significant changes as compared with non-reactive foods.

A major finding of this trial was that wheat, corn, and animal proteins were far more frequently reacting foods than vegetables or fruits (P < 0.0013).

I have only given a brief flavour of this trial, which in its original form is spread over 17 pages of close-printed A4 paper. I would recommend any physician interested in this subject to obtain the original, as it is full of excellent information and the tables detailing the changes that occurred in these patients between admission and discharge are truly impressive.

We now come to the British trial that was published in *The Lancet* in February 1986. The authors were Dr L.G. Darlington and Dr N.W. Ramsey of the Department of Rheumatology at Epsom District Hospital, and Dr J.R. Mansfield, The Burghwood Clinic, Banstead, Surrey. The trial was called 'A Placebo-controlled Blind Study of Dietary Manipulation Therapy in Rheumatoid Arthritis'. The aim of the study was to investigate as objectively as possible the effects of dietary elimination and challenge in patients with definite or classical rheumatoid arthritis. It will be noted that in this trial we did not take account of possible problems with chemicals, inhalants or candidiasis. Before we commenced the trial we had taken the problem to Dr J.R. Kirwan of the Bone and Joint Research Unit at the London Hospital for his advice about how to conduct the trial. Dr Kirwan is a leading authority on trial design and he suggested the following protocol.

A total of 53 patients (43 female, 10 male) entered the study as out-patients. They underwent a two-week washout period during which all previous therapy was withdrawn and they received only two placebo capsules (containing inert barium sulphate) with two paracetamol tablets four times daily. They were at this time taking their normal diets. The patients were then allocated randomly, either to immediate diet therapy (group B) or to a further six weeks of placebo therapy (group C) before then also proceeding to the diet therapy.

Trial design

During the first week of the diet, only foods of which the patient

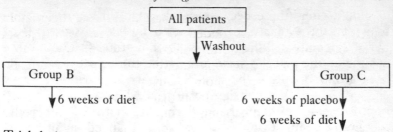

Trial design

was likely to be tolerant were given to allow other foods to be removed from the body. Other foods were then reintroduced one at a time to see whether symptoms were produced by dietary challenge. At first, further foods unlikely to cause intolerance were reintroduced, then foods such as cereals which often cause intolerance, then the remaining foods of a normal diet. We arranged reintroduction of foods from the same family more than four days apart to avoid complicating responses. After challenge any foods producing symptoms were excluded from the diet.

The aim of this unusual trial design (checked by two medical statisticians and one trial design specialist) was to maximize the chance of detecting spontaneous improvement and placebo response, and to make possible between-group and within-group comparisons. A cross-over design is not practical since many patients who have experienced symptoms with dietary challenge are unwilling to return to the previous diet. The study was single blind, since patients on dietary therapy cannot be blind to their treatment. Assessments were undertaken by a trained observer (Dr Ramsey) unaware of whether the patient was on dietary or placebo treatment or of the patient's stage of treatment. The clinical assessments were of pain by day and by night (on a four-point scale); average pain during 24 hours on a 10cm linear visual analogue scale; duration of morning stiffness; grip strength; the number of painful joints (detected by manual pressure by the same observer each time); and the time taken to walk 20 yards (18 metres). Laboratory measurements carried out were haemoglobin, absolute eosinophil count, platelet count, erythrocyte sedimentation rate, antinuclear antibodies, rheumatoid factor, C3, cryoglobulins, and fibrinogen. Details of the statistical analysis can be found in the original paper.

Results

Four patients defaulted too early for analysis and four others defaulted later (three because of uncontrolled arthritic symptoms). Of the 49 analysed, 48 completed week 1; in group B 24 out of 25 completed the full study; and in group C 23 out of 24 completed the placebo stage and 21 the full study.

In group B during the week of dietary elimination therapy eight variables changed significantly, of which seven indicated improvement. For comparison, during the first week of placebo therapy in group C only two variables changed significantly, showing improvement. During the full six weeks of dietary therapy in group B seven variables changed significantly, all indicating improvement, whereas during the full six weeks of placebo therapy in group C, three variables changed significantly, all denoting improvement.

When the dietary and placebo groups were compared the dietary group did better for all 13 variables for which differences between them were significant. Comparison of groups B and C while both were on dietary treatment showed only one significant difference. Comparison of placebo and diet periods in group C revealed benefit for the diet period for all 12 variables for which differences were significant.

When the patients had completed the dietary treatment, they were asked for their opinion of their response on a five-point scale 'much better' to 'much worse': 33 patients replying 'better' or 'much better' were considered to be good responders and 11 who replied 'the same', 'worse', or 'much worse' were poor responders. There were too few poor responders for separate analysis.

When we analysed the results in the same way for good responders only, the beneficial effect of the dietary manipulation was even more pronounced. During dietary therapy in group B 20 of 22 variables showing significant change denoted improvement; the corresponding numbers in group C were 14 of 14 variables. Comparisons between and within groups also significantly favoured the dietary group.

In summary we stated that in a blind, placebo-controlled study of dietary manipulation therapy in out-patients with rheumatoid arthritis there was significant objective improvement during periods of dietary therapy compared with periods of placebo therapy, particularly amongst 'good responders'.

We are of course looking forward to more trials performed in other units to further confirm these results. It will need many more trials of a similar nature before the medical profession will universally accept these ideas.

13   Clinical trials of neutralization

There have been a large number of clinical trials carried out in the USA and two in the UK. These trials were carried out on patients with a variety of symptom problems that appeared to be related to food or inhalant allergies. These included migraine, colitis, asthma, and rhinitis, as well as arthritis. One of the American trials had a lot of arthritic patients in it and one of the British trials had a few. I think, however, that it is reasonable to assume that if the adverse effects of a food allergen can be neutralized, it does not really matter which symptoms the food is causing. Certainly this is the common experience and this also applies to inhalant allergens.

Intradermal testing and neutralization

The first clinical trial to demonstrate the validity of neutralization therapy was organized by Dr Joseph Miller of Mobile, Alabama. The trial was published in *The Annals of Allergy*, Vol. 38, No. 3, March 1977, and entitled 'A Double-blind Study of Food Extract Injection Therapy'. Dr Miller was, as described earlier, the physician most connected with clarifying, organizing, and teaching this concept in the first place.

Patients who were selected for this study had illnesses strongly suspected to be caused by food sensitivity. Each of them was extensively tested for all the commonly-eaten foods by intradermal provocative neutralization testing. The neutralizing doses of the implicated foods were combined into a single injection solution specifically for each individual. The injections were self-administered subcutaneously daily for 20 days. Patients were restricted to eating those foods that had been assessed.

Placebo injections were prepared which were indistinguishable from the injections containing the active neutralizing doses. The placebo injections were also self-administered daily for 20 days. The first series of injections to be used (active or placebo) was decided randomly by the toss of a coin by a third party. Thus, neither the patient nor the physician was aware of which extracts were used. This trial, therefore, qualifies for the title of a double-blind trial. In the summary it was stated that the superiority of active extract over placebo extract for the eight patients involved was clearly significant at a 99.8 per cent level of confidence. In most patients the active extract was rapidly and markedly effective and the placebo was totally ineffective.

Case no. 1, for example, was a 29-year-old with severe migraine problems recurrent since early childhood, becoming progressively worse. In the preceding six months the headaches had awoken her in the early morning every day. She reported that headaches followed the ingestion of coffee, chocolate, beef, pork, and ice cream amongst other things. She had been taking potent drugs by mouth and potent injections for nine years. Additional symptoms included recurrent vertigo, buzzing in the ears, nausea, abdominal cramps, and depression.

The first series of injections administered was of active extract. After the third injection she required no further medication and was completely free of headache, vertigo, tinnitus and depression for the remainder of the 20 days. She stated that this was the longest period she had ever gone without a headache in her entire life. The nausea and abdominal cramps were present very mildly.

During the second series of injections (placebo) the headaches and all her other symptoms returned on the fourth day and remained severe for the rest of the 20 days. On the third series of injections (active) her symptoms had almost cleared by the third day and she remained virtually symptom-free for the rest of the 20–day period. On the fourth series (placebo) her symptoms returned again but not as severely as on the second series. This is a common finding in this type of trial. By the time the second placebo phase has started, the patient has had 40 desensitizing injections during the two active phases and the patient is beginning to become desensitized. This desensitizing effect carries over into the placebo phase, despite discontinuation of the active injections and provides some carry-over protection. Although this is evidence that a long-term desensitization effect occurs, it tends to diminish the difference between the active and placebo phases and thus understates the advantage of the active extract.

Another case in this study was also a severe migraine sufferer. She had had severe migraine accompanied by nausea and vomiting since early childhood which had become progressively worse in the seven months prior to the study. She had been awakened by severe headaches every morning at 4 o'clock. She had very frequent injections of narcotics such as pethidine in high dosage. Every three weeks or so these injections failed her and she was hospitalized and heavily sedated for three to seven days. She herself did not think it was likely that foods were related to her migraine.

The first series of injections (placebo) did not beneficially affect her at all. In the second series (active) the headaches became noticeably less severe after the third injection. Her photophobia and acne also became markedly better. Only a few mild headaches and one migraine occurred in the 20-day evaluation period. On the third series (placebo) she went rapidly downhill and by the sixth day her pethidine was no longer able to control her symptoms and she was re-admitted to hospital for five days. The headaches continued in their original severity and frequency for the rest of the 20 days. On the fourth series (active) she noticed improvement again on the fifth day and had no severe headaches for the rest of this phase.

In April 1984 Dr William J. Rea and his colleagues at the Environment Health Centre in Dallas reported a similar trial in *The Archives of Otolaryngology*, which was entitled 'Elimination of Oral Food Challenge Reactions by Ingestion of Food Extracts'. This trial was in my opinion attempting to do something rather more difficult than that which had been demonstrated in Dr Miller's trial. Dr Rea was attempting to turn off deliberately-induced food-allergic reactions with a single neutralizing dose of that food. As demonstrated in Dr Miller's trial, several sequential daily injections are often required before maximum benefit was obtained. I know this also from my own experience.

In their summary of the trial, the authors wrote that the results of this study were consistent with previous double-blind studies in providing support for the existence of the neutralizing dose effect that is different from and superior to the effect of the placebo. The responses in terms of signs and symptoms were divided into six possible variables. For each of these six variables a very significant difference was found between the neutralization and placebo situations. This demonstrated the effectiveness of the neutralizing dose in relief of symptomatology. The return of oral food challenge reactions when the placebo injections were used further emphasized the validity of the neutralizing dose method. Extremely elaborate precautions were taken to make these tests absolutely foolproof in terms of the double-blind, etc. and full details of this are given in the original paper. The paper concluded with the statement, 'It appears that the phenomenon of subcutaneous food neutralization can be scientifically endorsed for clinical use in the treatment of food reactions'.

Hyperactivity in children

Another study of neutralizing therapy was published in the *Journal of Learning Disabilities* in April 1984. The authors were Dr James O'Shea and Dr S.F. Porter. The purpose of the study was to determine by double-blind study whether the hyperkinetic syndrome (better known in Britain as hyperactivity) in children was at least partly due to individual reactions to foods, dyes, and inhalants. After being assessed by intradermal and sublingual testing, each patient was provided with composite individual extracts. As in Dr Miller's trial, an active phase and a placebo phase were employed. Each child's behaviour in each phase was monitored by parents, teachers, and a psychologist. Significant improvement was noticed in 11 out of the 14 children when treated with the active preparations as opposed to the placebos.

Inhaled allergy

In the field of inhaled allergy problems, there are as yet only three published trials relating to neutralization therapy. The first, by Drs Schiff, Weindorf, and Inselman, was published in *The Journal of Allergy and Clinical Immunology* in 1983. This trial was carried out entirely in the laboratory. The effect of neutralizing therapy on patients who had asthma induced by reactions to animal fur was evaluated using peak flow meters and other similar instruments.

All patients were first of all challenged with increasing amounts of animal dander until the amount required to cause a 20 per cent decrease in the peak flow was determined. Neutralizing levels were then obtained in the traditional way to the specific animal danders that were being used. The patients were given no treatment, placebo treatment, or active neutralization treatment. The results showed that the FEB 1 (force expiratory volume in one second) decreased 27.7 per cent from baseline in the controls, 25.9 per cent after placebo injections, but only 9.4 per cent after the active neutralizing injections. They concluded that there was a distinct diminution of animal dander-induced bronchospasm with neutralization therapy, which may well have important therapeutic implications.

These results are particularly good when it is considered that this improvement resulted from a single injection. As the previously-quoted trials have demonstrated, there is a build-up effect after several injections have been given.

Another trial, published in *Clinical Allergy* in 1986, was carried out at the Middlesex Hospital in London, by Dr Jonathan Brostoff and Dr Glenis Scadding of the Department of Immunology. They entitled the trial 'Low Dose Sublingual Therapy in Patients with Allergic Rhinitis due to House Dust Mite'. By low dose therapy they meant neutralization therapy. Summarizing their results, they stated that in a double-blind placebo-controlled cross-over trial, low dose sublingual therapy with house dust mite was effective in relieving symptoms in 72 per cent of the group of patients with perennial rhinitis due to house dust mite ($P < 0.03$). Following active treatment, there was a significant increase in morning peak nasal inspiratory flow rate ($P < 0.01$) in those who improved (13 out of 18) and resistance to nasal provocation with house dust mite also increased, in some cases up to 1000-fold ($P < 0.05$). The potential for oral desensitization is great and further studies of this form of treatment are needed.

Interestingly, if we analyse these results, we see that 13 out of 18 patients preferred the active preparation (the specific neutralizing dose) as their overall symptoms were improved by this treatment. However, 4 preferred the placebo (not because it provided any benefit, but because their symptoms were made worse by the active treatment). This would seem to mean that in four patients the neutralizing level on first assessment was incorrect. Re-testing will normally convert this situation into one of benefit. Only one patient was undecided and so was probably a genuine failure. Most patients in my experience have an even better response with neutralization for house dust mite administered by subcutaneous injection.

A further British trial was carried out at the Royal Liverpool Hospital under the guidance of my long-term friend and colleague, Dr Ronald Finn, who is a Consultant Physician at that hospital and an ex-President of the British Society for Allergy and Environmental Medicine. The trial was published in 1988 in the journal *Clinical Ecology*. The trial involved treatment programmes for both inhalant and food allergens.

To summarize the trial, it can be said that 53 patients with a variety of conditions were placed on a treatment programme comprising neutralization therapy plus selected environmental control. Overall there was a success rate of 66 per cent in a group of patients who had long-standing intractable disease. Most of the patients were secondary or tertiary referrals and had had so much medical attention that placebo effects were unlikely. Those patients who were highly allergic had a higher success rate (87 per cent) than the others, where the success rate was 44 per cent. Patients were considered highly allergic if their neutralizing levels were as low as No. 5. Patients with specific conditions, such as eczema, asthma and urticaria ($P < 0.05$), did better than other patients. Only 5 out of the 12 patients with arthropathy did well, which does not correlate with our own observations which would be much higher.

The authors conclude with the observation that these results are incompatible with a placebo effect or with a natural remission of the disease, and indicate that the overall success rate was due to a genuine effect of the treatment regime.

Sublingual provocation trials

There have been several reports relating to the efficacy and validity of sublingual testing for food allergies. These trials have not concerned themselves with the neutralization aspect, but have concentrated on whether patients can distinguish between a placebo and a sublingually-administered extract of a food to which they are sensitive. My view is that sublingual testing is markedly inferior to intradermal testing as it relies entirely on the patient's subjective response, both for diagnosis and for determination of the neutralizing level. The intradermal test has also the wheal appearance, indicating positivity or negativity, which is extremely helpful because, of course, it is independent of the patient's subjective feelings. Furthermore, I have the impression clinically that some foods are not absorbed well under the tongue and that this is a potent cause of inaccuracy. In 1981 *The Journal of Biological Psychiatry* published a paper by Dr D. King entitled 'Can Allergic Exposure Provoke Psychological Symptoms? A Double-blind Test'. This trial evaluated allergy patients who had at least one psychological symptom, such as anxiety, depression, confusion or problem with concentration. The question to be determined was, 'Did sublingual provocation with a specific food induce psychological symptoms more frequently than a placebo?' and 30 patients were challenged with selected foods and with triple-distilled water as a placebo. The trial was subdivided into four types of trial: (1) allergen trials — four allergy-producing foods each given three times; (2) placebo trials — two tests each given three times; (3) base rate trials in which the subjects received nothing sublingually but nevertheless received a complete evaluation; (4) open placebo trials to assess any biological reactivity of the placebo (three trials). Great care was taken to ensure that the test was properly double-blind, including the evaluation. Average symptom scores for psychological symptoms were four times higher after allergy-producing foods than after placebo provocation. The difference was highly statistically significant (P = 0.001). therefore Dr King would appear to have demonstrated that challenge sublingually with foods known to produce allergy can produce psychological symptoms much more frequently than placebo.

In July 1982 Dr Marshall Mandell and Dr A. Conte had a paper published in *The Journal of the International Academy of Preventive Medicine*. It was called 'The Role of Allergy in Arthritis, Rheumatism and Associated Polysymptomatic Cerebro-viscero-somatic Disorders: A Double-blind Provocation Test Study'. This study was initiated to determine the incidence and types of allergy present in arthritis and rheumatism and to confirm previous observations regarding the role of allergy in the causation of musculoskeletal disorders. Volunteers were tested for allergy and allergy-like sensitivities by a series of double-blind symptom-duplicating sublingual challenges with food extracts and other incitants including alternaria, house dust, tobacco smoke and petrochemicals (ethanol, natural gas, and car exhaust).

Many arthritic-rheumatic, cerebral, respiratory, vascular, gastrointestinal and eye reactions were induced in the 40 subjects. Test-evoked symptoms were identified by the subjects as their familiar chronic ailments. 'Rheumatic' joint and muscle reac-

tions, indistinguishable from presenting complaints, were induced in 35 (87.5 per cent of 40); nervous system reactions
(headache, restlessness, confusion, depression, itching, etc.)
were provoked in 38 (95 per cent) of the subjects. Respiratory,
vascular, gastrointestinal and eye symptoms were induced in 32
(80 per cent), 26 (65 per cent), 21 (52.5 per cent) and 16 (40 per
cent) of the subjects respectively.

This investigation demonstrated the importance of natural
and synthetic environmental incitants in the genesis of rheumatic syndromes. A comprehensive allergic-ecologic diagnosis was
indicated in each case. Ecologically orientated therapy may
eliminate or significantly reduce the need for symptom-
suppressing drugs that may cause avoidable, and perhaps
serious, side-effects.

It must be noted at this point that there have been two trials of
provocative sublingual testing which have shown totally negative
results. However, both trials were carried out in such a way that
a positive outcome was virtually impossible.

In 1980 *The Annals of Allergy* published a study by Dr C.
Lehman. He attempted to demonstrate whether sublingual food
challenges would induce changes in the oedema and swelling of
the mucous membrane of the nose and compared this with the
response to placebo drops. This study showed a totally negative
correlation, but the choice of one single parameter to measure
(i.e. the nasal mucous membrane) was a fundamental mistake.
In most clinical several clinical variables. As Dr Lehman himself
admitted, 'The nasal mucosal oedema is constantly changing at
10–minute intervals to other appearances quite independent of
whether foods or anything else are placed under the tongue'.

Thus the choice of such a fluctuating and unstable measure
invalidates any conclusion, positive or negative, that this trial
could produce. However, more important and in my view
amazingly, the patients were not even known to be allergic to the
specific foods that were tested. The subjects apparently only had
some 'history of food allergy'. Prior specific sensitivity was only
suspected for 11 out of the 60 foods that were challenged. This
makes the trial a complete nonsense, as for most of the time
patients' reactions to a food to which they were not even allergic
were being compared with a placebo.

The same sort of criticism applies to the 1973 report of the
Food Allergy Committee of the American Academy of Allergy.
Their subjects were supposed to have a 'known allergy to at least
one of the five foods to be surveyed', but the actual number who

were sensitive to each specific food was never reported. If, for example, each subject was actually sensitive to only one of the five test foods, a 20 per cent average response rate for food allergens would be expected. As there was a high placebo response rate in any case in this study, one would hardly expect a 20 per cent response rate to show any advantage over a placebo. There were in addition several other major omissions and methodological errors which completely, in my view, invalidated this report. Incredibly, only 3 out of the 10 participating physicians had any experience whatsoever with sublingual pro-vocation testing. It must be said that one is forced to wonder about the motivation of those involved in this trial.

Setting up clinical trials is a complex subject and needs to be done with great precision. Testing for food allergy needs a certain expertise, as do most medical tests. Those trials which have been reported by physicians who have been careful to take the precaution of precisely identifying specific food allergies and other similar extremely critical factors have all shown positive results for the identification of food sensitivities by sublingual testing. Thus, the results of the trials that have been done well have shown very positive proof that sublingual testing is valu-able.

In regard to the main factor, that is whether intradermal testing and neutralization is effective, there have been no published trials which one can set against the very positive results detailed earlier in this chapter. In 1987 a well-known allergist, Dr David Freed of Manchester University, published an extensive critique of all the evidence relating to intradermal testing and neutralization therapy. He concluded that the evidence was now strong. For years he had been very sceptical of this technique. He now uses it extensively himself and wishes he had used it much earlier.

14　The roots of allergy

The main factors at the root of the allergic problem appear to be: (1) basic nutritional deficiencies; (2) a monotonous, repetitive diet; (3) the chemical adulteration of food; (4) chronic intestinal thrush (candidiasis). This list is not in order of importance as I think that the chronic intestinal thrush is possibly the most important factor.

The effect that basic nutritional factors could have on animals (and hence man) was most brilliantly demonstrated in 1945 by what has been known as the Pottenger Cat Studies.

The Pottenger cat studies

Drug companies are well aware that in most respects cats respond similarly to human beings and so they are widely used for testing drugs. These experiments were suggested by Pottenger's observation that cats fed on a raw meat and untreated milk diet were much better operative risks than those fed cooked meat and untreated milk. In a series of experiments one group of cats was fed on a diet of two-thirds raw meat, one-third milk and cod-liver oil. A second group was fed on a diet of two-thirds cooked meat, one-third milk and cod-liver oil. Nine hundred cats were studied over a period of ten years.

The cats receiving raw meat reproduced normally, had few abortions, nursed their young well, had very good behaviour patterns and a high resistance to infections and parasites.

The cats receiving the cooked meat reproduced poorly in general and there was an abortion rate of 25 per cent in the first generation, increasing to 70 per cent in the second generation. Many cats died in labour and the mortality rate in the kittens was high. The cats were irritable and difficult to handle, skin lesions and allergies were frequent and became progressively worse from generation to generation while the cats remained on the same diet. In addition, the oral arches narrowed, and osteomyelitis, cardiac lesions, thyroid disease, nephritis, hepatitis, *arthritis*, and many other conditions familiar to human beings all became common. Of the cats maintained entirely on the cooked meat and milk diet, the kittens of the third generation were so degenerated that none of them survived the first six months of life, thereby terminating the strain.

Cats of the first and second generation cooked meat group were later returned to a raw meat diet. Of enormous significance was the fact that it took three to four generations before the offspring regained good health. At the beginning of this century people in the Western world started to eat highly refined and processed foods, with a high percentage of our food cooked. We are, therefore, in approximately the third or fourth generations of eating such foods and increasingly we are getting the same diseases that the cats did.

There follows from this work the enormous implication that a condition which may be currently considered genetic in origin could stem from poor nutrition in an earlier generation. The other, less happy implication is that really adequate nutrition may fail to correct chronic diseases within one generation. This is not to say, however, that allergy management could not do the same job.

This trial report is not a plea for human beings to exist entirely on raw food and milk! It is, however, a demonstration that inadequate nutrition can have a disastrous effect in terms of disease on one species and there is no reason to believe that inadequate diet could not have the same effect on human beings. Pottenger surmised that the problem could well be the denaturing of protein by heat. Certainly, heating meat alters its physiochemical state in the same way as processing other foods will alter their ability to remain perfect for the maintenance of health.

Basic nutritional deficiencies

In the past few years there has been an enormous upsurge in interest in the nutritional basis of disturbances of the immune system. There is no question that the immune system is involved with the engendering of arthritis and there is now no doubt that deficiencies or excesses of certain nutrients can have the most dramatic effects on the proper functioning of that system.

In Britain there is the British Society for Nutritional Medicine and a number of physicians and laboratories are busily identifying the nutritional status of individual patients. Once this has been done, measures can be taken to correct the deficiencies or excesses that are discovered. The laboratories can identify these problems by blood serum or hair analysis, and sweat test examinations, among other methods. It is my practice to refer for analysis arthritis patients who from preliminary investigation appear to have widespread immune dysfunction.

A monotonous, repetitive diet

Humans have eaten vegetables, fruit, fish and meat since the Stone Age. Physicians working with food-allergic patients know that these foods, especially in their organic form, are for most patients the safest. The reason for this is probably that we have, as a species, eaten these foods for two to three million years and we are hence fairly well adapted to them. Any of our forebears who could not tolerate these types of food have probably tended to die out. The Stone Age diet was conceived by Dr Richard Mackarness as a relatively safe diet on which many food-allergic patients would improve as it avoids all the common food allergens. A perusal of the food trials shows wheat to be the commonest item implicated with arthritis. Corn, milk, eggs, cane and beet sugar, yeast, and soya beans are also among the more common offenders.

Although bread is regarded by many people to be the 'staff of life', most people are surprised to learn that cereals such as wheat and corn are a relatively recent addition to the human diet. Corn was originally planted in Egypt 4,000 years ago, but there is no evidence of cereals being grown in Britain prior to the Roman invasion around 2,000 years ago. Yeast has probably been used for about 8,000 years, originally to make scrumpy. Sugar was unknown in Britain until cane sugar was brought from the West Indies in the sixteenth century, only about 400 years ago.

Soya beans have been introduced into Britain only since 1955. They now crop up in a multitude of ways, usually in the form of soya-bean oil or soya-bean flour. Soya-bean oil is found in many wholemeal breads. It is also present, usually vaguely labelled as vegetable oil, in margarine, ice cream, salad dressings, and mayonnaise. Soya-bean flour is also found in sausages, luncheon meats, and confectionery. Thus, most of our major foods have only been in our diet for a couple of hundred — or thousand — years and, in terms of evolution and adaptation, two thousand years is only yesterday.

In Chapter 9 I detailed the multitude of ways in which corn creeps into most people's everyday diet. Many people eat corn in over ten different ways every day of their life. The invention of complex food mixtures by the food industry has made it very easy to eat small amounts of wheat, corn, milk, eggs, soy, cane and beet sugar very frequently throughout the day. It would appear that this frequent 'peppering' of our enzyme systems by these foods is very important in the engendering of food sensitivity.

Part of the evidence for this is that it very frequently turns out that foods which people eat most frequently and addictively are the ones to which they are sensitive. Admittedly, by the time an individual is seen by the doctor, the addictive factor may be due to the allergy having developed.

Further evidence is provided by observations related to the development of tolerance to foods that at one time produced allergy. If an allergic food is left out of the diet for a period of between three months and two years, tolerance will develop in most instances. It is then observed that, if the food is only eaten about once every four or five days, this tolerance will be maintained. If the food is eaten more frequently, the tolerance is usually destroyed and an allergic response will again result. These observations are the basis of the rotation diet, which is often useful in the management of food allergies. The idea of such a diet is that no food is repeated more than once every four or five days. On such a diet new food allergies virtually never occur, but it is of course difficult to maintain socially. Nevertheless, the effectiveness of such regimes is further proof that the frequency with which a food is ingested is very important in the causation of allergy.

Chemicals in food and the environment

That chemicals can lead to allergic phenomena has already been described in Chapter 3. Chemicals are known not to be antigenic, but it is throught that some bind to proteins to form haptens (incomplete antigens). There is evidence to suggest furthermore that chemicals can contribute to making the mucous membranes of the intestines leaky. I have already dealt with this in greater detail in Chapter 6. In addition, it is likely that chemicals can lead to food susceptibility in terms of the load they create on the immune system.

Dr William Rea of the Brookhaven Medical Centre in Dallas recently invented the barrel concept of allergy. This illustrates the concept that various allergies can have a cumulative effect and, when enough of this effect occurs, the barrel overflows and symptoms result. I have seen many patients who will react to certain foods when in a polluted environment, but not when in a clean environment.

Chronic intestinal thrush (candidiasis)

This subject has already been discussed in Chapter 6. Here it is only described in the context in which it may dovetail with other basic causes of allergy. A few years ago, an article in *The Lancet* covered a controlled study indicating that patients with food or skin allergies had leaky mucous membranes which could admit many more protein molecules than was normal. Patients thus developed multiple food and chemical sensitivities because antibodies were formed to the antigenic proteins in food, pollens, and even their own microbiological flora of the gut. This flora includes fungi, such as Candida, trichophyton and epidermophyton. Mucous membranes can also be made to leak by excessive exposure to toxic chemicals and almost certainly by the sort of nutritional deficiencies which have been described earlier in this chapter.

The critical mechanisms underlying the whole food and chemical allergy problem are therefore probably related to leaky mucous membranes in the intestine and these are in turn caused by the various factors which have been discussed in this chapter. Some of these factors may be more important in some patients than in others. My opinion, based on general experience of dealing with patients rather than hard clinical data, is that the Candida problem is probably the most significant. Very likely in many patients these factors interweave to produce the final result. Quite probably, once the situation occurs in which the development of food sensitivity is likely, repeated ingestion of a certain food which is new to our diet will then make it further likely that an allergy will develop.

Resistance and adaptation

Up to now I have dwelt almost exclusively on the various factors that constitute the insult to the host, that is, the individual. As with all equations, however, the final result depends on the interplay of two factors: (1) the nature of the insult or attack on the host; (2) the resistance and natural adaptive resources of the host.

The work that has most clarified this aspect was done by Hans Selye, the eminent physiologist, working in his laboratory at the University of Montreal. Selye's work on what is termed 'the general adaptation syndrome' will almost certainly eventually rank among the greatest medical discoveries of all time: he has clarified the mechanisms of adaptation to stress. This does not just mean psychological stress but, also and more importantly, the struggle of the human body to stay healthy in the face of the whole gamut of potentially harmful agents with which it is in daily contact. Selye has defined stress as the rate at which wear and tear is induced in the body by the process of living.

It is now known that cortisone, which is produced by the cortex of our adrenal glands, is our main defence against allergic reactions of all types. Selye was the first to demonstrate that cortisone had a protective effect and was also able to mobilize the body's other defences against allergic reactions and other harmful events. In 1936 Selye published a letter in the journal *Nature* entitled, 'A Syndrome Produced by Diverse Nocuous Agents'. The letter starts as follows:

Experiments on rats show that, if the organism is severely damaged by acute, non-specific noxious agents, such as exposure to cold, surgical injury, excessive muscular exercise or intoxications with sublethal doses of diverse drugs, a typical syndrome appears, the symptoms of which are independent of the nature of the damaging agent or the pharmacological type of drug employed and represent rather a response to damage as such.

Later in the latter Selye describes the three stages of the general adaptation syndrome. Stage 1 (the alarm reaction) started about 6 to 48 hours after the initial injury. It is akin to what most doctors refer to as surgical shock and is characterized by low blood pressure, loss of muscle tone, and shrinkage of the adrenal glands as they pump out as much cortisone as possible. There were also other symptoms, such as leakage of fluid from the smaller blood vessels into the surrounding tissues.

Stage 2 started about 48 hours after the original injury. There was now considerable enlargement of the adrenal glands and the swelling in the tissues, produced by the leakage of fluid from the blood vessels, started to subside. The pituitary gland, which controls virtually all the other glands in the body, produced increased amounts of a hormone (adreno-cortico-stimulating hormone) which in turn caused the adrenal glands to produce more cortisone.

When further small repeated doses of the harmful stimulus were given, be it an allergy-producing stimulus or any other, the rats built up a resistance. Hence they had become adapted and in this phase they outwardly showed no symptoms at all.

If the rats in this adapted stage were removed from the harmful stress, for example the persistent cold stimulus, it was found that they lost their newly-acquired resistance to the cold within a few days. When reintroduced to the cold environment they had to go through the Stage 1 alarm reaction. Conversely, if the rats were left in the cold, they continued adapting for a long time, apparently having grown completely used to it.

This is of course what has been described earlier in the book in Chapter 2 in the section about masking to foods. This mechanism of masking represents the continued application of the harmful stimulus and the body's adapted response to it. The exaggerated adverse response (Rinkel's hyperacute response), when the body was re-exposed to that food after a period (five days plus) of avoiding it, is a Stage 1 alarm reaction.

If the rats continued to be exposed for a long time to the cold stimulus they seemed at first to be perfectly well, but after a period of time they became ill and eventually died. They had entered a stage of maladaption and eventually a stage of exhaustion. The symptoms in this Stage 3 (maladaption and then exhaustion) were similar to Stage 1 (the alarm stage). In Stage 3 only complete removel of the harmful stimulus would produce a healthy animal. The transition from the adapted to the maladapted/exhaustion stage is clinically known as the start of the current illness.

Why someone goes from the adapted phase to the non-adapted phase is not always obvious. In some people there appears to be no particular reason why arthritis should start at a particular age. Maybe the body is just becoming older and less able to keep up successful adaptation. In other cases it appears obvious that 'the straw that broke the camel's back' was an event that produced a temporary excessive stress on the system. In many people arthritis starts soon after a severe attack of flu, glandular fever, or a similar virus illness. Childbirth, major operations, and accidents are physically stressful events which can also be the 'final straw'.

Major psychological stresses can also have the same effect. In a recent study published in the USA it was shown that bereavement caused a diminution in the T-lymphocyte count in most people. The level of the T-lymphocytes is possibly one of the better indications of the competence of the immune system to deal with allergic phenomena.

There is a condition called myalgic encephalomyelitis (ME), or 'Royal Free disease', which is a severe meningitis-like illness. In a high proportion of cases, after they recover from the primary illness they are never the same again. Many suffer from a wide range of symptoms: fatigue, depression, headaches, nausea and so on. I have treated a lot of these patients and most of these symptoms are related to food allergy or intestinal thrush and can be eradicated by dealing with these particular problems. I am sure, therefore, that in these people the severe viral illness was just a major stressful event which cause them to start to react to dormant food allergies or thrush.

Thus, people start to react to foods in the middle part of their lives because of their failure to maintain their adaptation to them. Foods which had appeared to be perfectly innocuous for often twenty to forty years suddenly become harmful. The whole root of the arthritis problem can thus be summarized by Figure 5.

Although everything in this diagram is, I believe, basically valid and there is much evidence to support it, there is an awful lot that we still do not know. Most problems can have an explanation at various levels. I have sought to explain this disease in terms of the aggravating or 'insulting' factors and the adaptive reactions of the individual to these. This might be described as the macro-reaction. The micro-reaction, that is the particulars of the cellular or immunological response, are not at all well understood at the present time. The immunologic reaction to most foods is totally unknown. Although a few food reactions are modulated by immunoglobulin E (IgE) the vast majority are not. It is though that immunoglobulin G, perhaps IgG 4, may be the one that is involved in most food-allergic reactions, but this is pure speculation at the moment. As discussed in Chapter 10, we do know some details of how a reaction which starts as an allergy can then become an inflammation (see page 139).

The fact that we do not yet understand the immunological

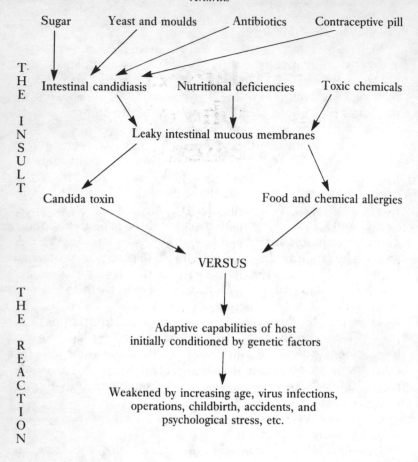

Figure 5 The interrelationship of Candida, allergy and arthritis

response, however, does not mean that we cannot adequately deal with the condition. It could well be fifty years before the details of the immunological response are finally identified. In the meantime, there are millions of arthritis patients who can be helped and often completely cured by the knowledge that is currently available.

15 The language and philosophy of New Medicine

The way that illness is described and the perception of such illness by doctors is very much tied up with the problem of achieving general recognition and acceptance of this approach by the medical profession at large. The mental re-orientation needed by most doctors to understand and appreciate the significance of this subject is quite enormous as it implies going back to square one and starting again in terms of their medical philosophy. This is not easy for conservative people used to diligently travelling in one direction for most of their career. Many physicians find these concepts both challenging and somewhat alarming to their established order of life. Some, therefore, to the consternation of their patients, react with distinct aggression to these concepts. Two consultant rheumatologists have told me that they were glad that they were soon retiring and hence would not have to rethink their whole approach to their job.

Most major changes in medical thought and direction have always taken about 30–50 years to become generally accepted. Minor changes such as a new anti-inflammatory drug are in contrast accepted very quickly. The germ theory, for example, was ridiculed by the medical profession in the last century before it became medical orthodoxy over 30 years after its initial discovery. Other major discoveries, like Harvey's 'circulation of the blood', had similar problems with recognition.

The new approach to illness described in this book in relation to arthritis has implications throughout the realm of chronic illness. The subject has been termed variously as Allergy, Environmental Medicine, Clinical Ecology, Nutriallergy, etc. but none of these terms are by themselves sufficiently wide to embrace the whole field and communicate exactly what we do to either the medical profession or the medical consuming public.

The name of the society of British physicians involved in this subject has become the British Society for Allergy and Environmental Medicine and this term is probably as good as any immediately available.

Names, though, are important and in medicine very important, as witness the battles relating to the terms allergy, intolerance and hypersensitivity. Names do also condition the way that we think about illness and also the way that we deal with it.

The language of illness

When we think of illness we usually think of specific disease entities and these are called diagnoses. A diagnosis ideally tells a lot about an illness. Various acute diseases such as measles lend themselves particularly well to this idea. The term 'measles' tells us which micro-organism is causing the problem, the incubation period of the disease, the type of rash that occurs, how long the rash will last, the likely complications and so on. This same diagnostic philosophy also works well with chickenpox, polio, mumps, whooping cough, etc. Diagnosis is supposed to be aetiologic, that is to explain the cause, and in the examples given above it does this very satisfactorily.

The specific diagnosis idea, however, works less well with a diagnosis like bronchitis. Bronchitis is an inflammation of the bronchial tubes in the chest, but this inflammation can be caused by a wide variety of different germs. Furthermore, the condition occurs only in certain people who are susceptible to the disease, and this susceptibility can be heightened by environmental factors such as cigarette smoking and industrial pollution. Therefore one cannot say that any particular germ is the cause of the problem, or necessarily that it is the cigarette smoking, the industrial pollution, or the individual susceptibility of the host. To say, therefore, that bronchitis causes symptoms of wheezing and coughing is not strictly true.

When we come to most chronic diseases the 'status and value' of the diagnosis becomes even less significant. This particularly applies to conditions like arthritis. Patients are asked by their physicians to accept the idea that the pain and stiffness in their joints is caused by arthritis, which is untrue as symptoms are not caused by the process named, as in the bronchitis example. Some doctors might reasonably argue that as the 'cause' of arthritis is not known (in their view), such naming performs all the function needed of a diagnostic term. However, talking about the disease as a cause of symptoms leads to treating the disease rather than the person who is ill. The tendency for doctors to speak and act as if they are treating diseases, not individuals, and the implication that people become ill because they are hapless victims are two of the most important issues that lie embedded in medical language.

Let us now return to matters discussed earlier. We have seen that individual adverse reactions to foodstuffs, chemicals, inhalant particles, and the flora of the gut can produce widely varying symptoms in different individuals, as illustrated by four well-documented medical statements:

1. 'Milk Sensitivity Can Produce Rheumatoid Arthritis' Park, A. C. and Hughes, G. R. V., Rheumatoid Arthritis and Food – A Case Study, *British Medical Journal*, 1981, 282, pp 2027–2029.

2. 'Milk Allergy Can Produce Ulcerative Colitis in 20% of Cases with Ulcerative Colitis' Professor Truelove, *British Medical Journal*, 1962.

3. 'Milk Allergy Can Produce Eczema – A Double-blind Controlled Crossover Trial of Antigen Avoidance Diet in Atopic Eczema' D. J. Atherton and J. F. Soothill, *Lancet*, 25th February, 1978.

4. 'Milk Allergy Can Produce Migraine – Is Migraine Food Allergy?' Soothill et al., *Lancet*, October, 1983.

Thus, adverse reactions to milk can masquerade as a wide variety of symptoms in different people. Similar multiple masquerades can be shown by other foods, chemicals and inhalants, etc. The different guises that reactions to individual items can manifest is most practical reason for developing a system of describing signs and symptoms in individuals that should give us a basis for learning about and treating illness that transcends just naming and treating the symptoms.

The crux of the difference between treating the individual and treating the diagnostic label lies mostly in the consideration given to symptoms that may seem superfluous to a particular diagnosis.

Symptoms like fatigue, headache, wind, bloating, palpitations, food addiction, excessive sweating, weight gain, adverse responses to alcohol, and anal irritation, to name but a few, are quite extraneous in orthodox medicine to making the diagnosis of rheumatoid arthritis, osteoarthritis, non-specific arthritis, gout, or psoriatic arthritis. However, as discussed earlier, they are very useful when we are looking at the base causes of joint pain, swelling, and stiffness. In fact they are possibly more useful than those features of the patient's history and examination which cause us to label them as suffering from these varying types of arthritis.

Professor Sidney Baker, who is Research Director of the Gessell Institute of Human Development in Newhaven, Connecticut, has been at the forefront of medical thinking in this area. He has proposed a highly elaborate three-dimensional matrix computer programme which will enable physicians to enter all of the sorts of information I have alluded to, to provide an enormous database for progress in this subject. Currently it is being used by all the physicians within the Medical Department of the Gessell Institute, and by the time this book is published a number of other physicians in the United States will be involved also. Ultimately it is expected that over 100 physicians will collaborate.

One way of illustrating the masquerades these various environmental agents can take is to take various classical disease entities and to describe the role that certain basic causes play in these specific entities. Some of these 'contributions' have been established in published clinical trials, but many of these associations have been noted by physicians working in the field and used as part of their daily practice. In Figure 6, uninterrupted lines indicate a relationship shown in a published clinical trial; interrupted lines show associations that have been observed but not as yet verified by formal clinical trials.

The lines in the lower part of these diagrams joining the various causes of diseases are entirely based on the clinical experience of physicians and their observations. For instance, the chemical sensitivity usually diminishes or disappears after treatment for Candida. Also, of course, Candida is usually connected with nutritional factors such as high sugar consumption.

Thus it is emerging that almost any chronic disease can have almost any cause and almost any cause can lead to almost any condition. The logical way of dealing with these problems is therefore to diagnose which particular causative factor(s) could be relevant in each particular patient. The techniques are of course those described in this book.

Physicians who like to view disease in terms of cause and

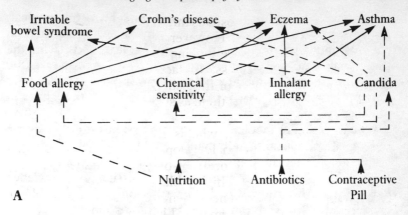

A

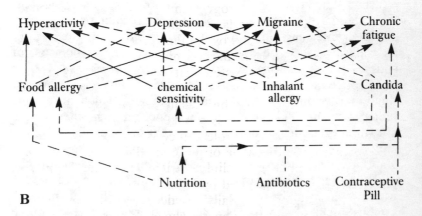

B

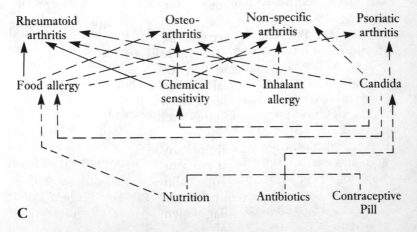

C

Figure 6 Interrelationships of cause and effects

effect have been naturally drawn, like myself, to this subject. Many other doctors are, however, uneasy when looking at patients and medicine from this point of view and prefer the traditional organ-based approach. In fact, for well over 2,000 years the history of medicine has demonstrated this constant schism between the two major directions of thought and philosophy.

One direction of medical thought can best be described as the rationalist school, and at the moment this school of thought dominates the teaching at medical schools throughout most of the world. This school prefers the approach of knowledge derived from the study of pathology (the study of organs, blood, etc.) followed by symptom suppression, for example by the use of drugs. The other direction is the empirical school of thought. This approach is based on the observation of patients' symptoms and their interreaction with the environment, using the term in its widest sense. The approach described in this book is, of course, of the empirical school.

Throughout medical history these two main currents of thought have flowed their separate courses, which have conflicted with and yet have exerted influence on each other. There are some examples of empirical thought in rationalist teaching and vice versa. Certainly the rationalist approach has brought about many major advances in medicine but the biggest advance of all, the germ concept of disease, was initially an empirical idea which was strongly resisted for many years by the medical establishment of the day. Bacteria and viruses are of course external environmental agents and their effect on human beings is now well accepted.

Sir Francis Bacon, who was a founder of modern science and an empiricist, believed that the purpose of science was to observe, describe, and characterize the processes of nature, rather than necessarily to explain them. Hippocrates made the empirical observation that certain people were harmed by eating cheese, but most are not. Therefore there must be something in the reactivity of the individual rather than in the cheese itself. This conflicted with a tendency of most physicians of the rationalist school initiated by Aristotle to prefer pathological knowledge over symptomatic observations, ignoring symptoms unless they happened to fit in with their preconceived concepts.

My rationalist medical school education taught me to focus my attention on to specific disease entities and on pathological findings, especially objective laboratory findings. It was necessary to find something wrong with the patient with objective tests in order to have a 'rational basis for treatment'. The treatment then took the direction of opposing, combating, or suppressing symptoms with analgesic drugs, anti-spasmodic drugs, anti-inflammatory drugs, anti-arthritic drugs, and so on.

In the last century Constantine Hering taught that the suppression of acute illness tends to promote chronic illness. He also taught that the natural processes of healing functioned best when the physician promoted the reversion of chronic symptoms to acute symptoms. In this respect Hering foresaw the basic concept of our approach; that a return to health requires an initial clearing of the chronic adaptive state (as, for example, on the five- to six-day hypoallergenic diet) after which time chronic symptoms can revert to acute symptoms (Rinkel's hyperacute response). At this stage the various excitants can be identified.

Most physicians, because of the training which directs their attention, belief and behaviour on the rationalist approach, find it difficult to accept empirical approaches and regard them as unscientific or not being within the scope of the practice of medicine.

An example of this is the role of cigarette smoking in the causation of lung cancer, a classic instance of an environmental stimulus causing a disease process. In 1958 I was a medical student and, having reviewed all the clinical papers supporting this view, I discussed the matter with several consultants at my medical school. In view of the weight of evidence I wanted to know why the fact that cigarette smoking was a cause of lung cancer was not at that time being taught at my medical school. I was told that, if I believed that cigarette smoking was a cause of lung cancer, I was mad. That lung cancer could be caused by an environmental agent such as a simple cigarette was beyond belief. These physicians were much more interested in teaching the various histological forms that cancer could take rather than the environmental agents that could cause it.

In fact there is an inherent desire in most scientists to prefer complex research to simple research. They would argue that only by complex research into the intricate details of bodily functions can we gain an overall picture of disease processes and only then can we succeed in combating disease. Such an argument has inherent flaws. In most cases bodily mechanisms are so complex that it will take many decades or many centuries to understand them properly. The problem is similar to an underground system of such vastness that as soon as one channel is charted two or three new ones are discovered. This rationalist-inspired complex research is therefore likely to be a very long-term saga with no guarantee of anything useful emanating at the end of it. Simple research into the interrelationship of lung cancer and cigarette smoking has yielded enormous practical benefits in indicating the value of stopping this habit. Many thousands of lives have already been saved as a result of this research.

In contrast to the above, complex research such as gene regulation of the metabolism of thousands of chemicals in tobacco smoke and their effect on the human body has been of minute value.

One of the interesting things about medicine is that it is often hard to establish the specific time that a new concept has become generally acceptable. In which year, for example, was it finally accepted that cigarette smoking was the main cause of lung cancer? Possibly about five years ago, as I do not remember any concerted arguments to the contrary being advanced in the last five years. There is in truth no particular point in time. As Dr Ronald Finn once told me, there are four stages in the development of a new medical idea:

Stage 1: You are mad.
Stage 2: I suppose there might be something in it.
Stage 3: There could be something in it, but where is the proof?
Stage 4: Well, of course we knew all along.

Dr Finn thinks that we are in Stage 3 at the moment in regard to the environmental view of medicine. However, because of all these conflicting outlooks it may be quite a long time before this approach is available in all clinics and hospitals, despite the positive evidence. There is no disadvantage in terms of cost in this approach to arthritis, as it is indeed highly cost-effective. Four or five consultations and a couple of skin-testing sessions will often obviate the need for repeated consultations extending over 20 or more years and constant drugging with anti-inflammatory and disease-modifying drugs. There is of course also the enormous economic advantage of patients able to continue in gainful employment and not being an economic burden to the community.

I would like to thank Dr Karl Humiston of New York for some of the source material for this chapter.

Summary

This book has described a revolutionary new approach to the management of most forms of arthritis, based entirely on trying to determine cause and effect as opposed to straightforward symptom suppression. This approach started several years ago with the observation that food sensitivities were important and seemed to be major factors in the aetiology of this condition in certain patients.

These observations were to a large extent confirmed by the clinical trial that my clinic performed in conjunction with the Department of Rheumatology at Epsom District Hospital and which was later published in *The Lancet* in February 1986. In that trial we showed that 75 per cent of 44 patients improved considerably or entirely on an elimination diet compared with only one or two on placebo treatment. A similar trial published in the USA gave similar but better results as environmental factors were taken into account as well.

Dr Theron Randolph of Chicago, Illinois, has brought to our attention the fact that chemical sensitivity is important in many patients with arthritis, and this realization has led to further patients having the cause of their problems identified.

Other physicians came to realize that allergic reactions to house dust, dust mites, moulds, and other similar inhaled particles could not only produce symptoms of catarrh and asthma, but could also be major contributing factors in the production of this disease. Neutralization treatment is the only practical way, short of emigration to a hot dry climate, that can deal with this type of problem.

The work of Dr Orion Truss, which showed that intestinal candidiasis could cause symptoms in bodily systems outside the digestive tract, has led to further patients being relieved of their arthritic symptoms who would otherwise have been regarded as treatment failures.

In other parts of this book I have discussed the whole nutritional basis of allergy and of intestinal candidiasis. Candidiasis appears to be a major cause of chemical sensitivity and almost certainly of multiple food sensitivity. Thus all these factors are interrelated and the complex web of effects that they produce between them can lead to problems such as joint pain, swelling and stiffness.

Whether these joint problems are labelled rheumatoid arthritis, osteoarthritis, non-specific arthritis or psoriatic arthritis does not appear to matter when we are talking about the causative factors, because all of them seem to respond similarly to this type of investigation.

For those people whose problem is straightforward food sensitivity there is a description of how an elimination diet can be utilized to isolate these sensitivities. I hope this information will be valuable to physicians who wish to explore the subject with their own patients.

There are several chapters on the technique and uses of neutralization therapy, essentially to give an idea of the scope and value of this technique. Any physician becoming seriously interested in the technique would be advised to obtain Professor J.B. Miller's original book on the subject and obtain practical instruction, either by attending the many courses held each year in the United States or by visiting clinics familiar with this technique in the United Kingdom. I have included a chapter detailing trials that have validated this technique.

The problems of recognition were explored in the last chapter. Several thousand patients in the UK alone have already had their joint problems reversed, sometimes in as short a period of time as a few weeks. Many physicians have been impressed by these recoveries and a few rheumatologists are now following this same path. Interesting one doctor after another is, however, a painfully slow method of disseminating this type of knowledge. Both our *Lancet*-published trial and the American trial produced little reaction from the medical establishment and I know of only one other clinical trial in progress in the United Kingdom at the moment attempting to verify our findings.

Millions of people in Britain alone suffer from arthritis to a greater or lesser extent and the effect both economically and in sheer human suffering is incalculable. What I would like is a major investigation into this approach by a body such as the

Medical Research Council, guided by physicians already familiar with the subject. These findings need to be validated as a matter of urgency and validated to the extent that they can be taught in medical school and become part of mainstream medicine.

As with many discoveries in life, the biggest problem is not really in making the actual discovery, but in its dissemination and recognition. Are the methods of human communication so inadequate that a method of curing one of the most crippling diseases known to mankind is discovered, used successfully in a large number of patients, written about extensively, and yet remains unknown to most of the medical profession and most patients who suffer the condition? Hence this book, which I hope will go some way to rectify this situation.

Useful addresses

Many of these are voluntary groups, funded by donations. When writing to them, please enclose a large, stamped self-addressed envelope to save them time and money.

Action Against Allergy
43 The Downs
London SW20 8HG
Telephone: 01-947 5082
(Mrs A. Nathan-Hill)

Allergy Support Group, Oxford
36 Blandford Avenue
Oxford
Telephone: (0865) 58931
(Mrs V. Hibbert)

Cambridge Food Intolerance Society
1 Gunhild Close
Cambridge
Telephone: (0223) 240895
(Mrs B. Stone)

Chemical Victims
12 Highlands Road
Worting
Nr Basingstoke
Hants
Telephone: (0256) 65093
(Mrs S. Hedges)

The Fighting Food Allergy Group
Little Porters
64a Marshals Drive
St Albans
Herts
Telephone: (0727) 58705
(Chrys Dowsett)

Food and Chemical Allergy Association
27 Ferringham Lane
Ferring-by-Sea
West Sussex
Telephone: (0903) 41178
(Mrs E. Rothera)

Hythe Food and Chemical Victims' Allergy Club
44 Fairview Drive
Hythe
Southampton
(Mr J. Spells)
No telephone enquiries

National Society of Research into Allergy
P.O. Box 45
Hinkley
Leicester LE10 1JY
Telephone: (0455) 635212
(Mrs E. Rose)

Seaford Food and Chemical Group
57 Sutton Grove
Seaford
Sussex BN25 3NQ
Telephone: (0323) 893779
(Mrs R. Jones)

West Sussex Allergy Group
28 The Avenue
Chichester
West Sussex PO19 4PU
Telephone: (0243) 527321
(Mrs A. Shapiro)

Irish Allergy Association
P.O. Box 1067
Churchtown
Dublin 14

The Human Ecology Research Foundation
505 North Lake Shore Drive
Suite 6506
Chicago, Illinois 60611, USA

Alan Mandell Center for Bio-Ecologic Diseases
3 Brush Street
Norwalk, Connecticut 06850, USA

American Academy of Environmental Medicine
1750 Humboldt Street
Denver, Colorado 80218, USA

Allergy Association of Australia
P.O. Box 298
Ringwood
Victoria 3134
Australia
Telephone: 03 720 3215

Allergy and Intolerant Reactions Association
P.O. Box 1780
Canberra City 2601
Australia

Allergy Recognition and Management
P.O. Box 2
Sandy Bay
Tasmania 7005
Telephone: 002 236 797

Allergy Awareness Association
P.O. Box 120701
Penrose
Auckland 6
New Zealand

Index

acupuncture 41-2
adaptation 27-8, 172-6
addiction to foods 53, 56-7, 104
  and masked food allergy 25-6
additives, chemical 46-8
alcohol 52-5, 104, 125
  constituents of 54-5
  rapid absorption of 52-3
alcoholism and food allergy 53-4
allergy
  defining 22-4
  intolerance 9
  roots of 168-76
  tests for 35-40
  see also food allergy
American Academy of
  Environmental Medicine 35
Amphotericin-B 70, 77-8, 80
animal dander 37, 58, 63, 117, 145,
  162-3
ankylosing spondylitis 19-20, 90-2,
  96-7
Annals of Allergy 21, 150, 159, 166
anti-Candida diet 71-4, 86, 87, 88
anti-inflammatory drugs 62, 95
antibiotics 66, 68, 69, 77-8
applied kinesiology 38-9
Archives of Otolaryngology 161
aspirin 13, 109
asthma 25, 58, 105, 131-2, 133, 159,
  162, 164
auto-immune urine therapy 41
auto-immunity 10-11
avoidance of foods, difficulty of 141,
  171

Baker, Professor Sidney 180
basophils 137, 138
benzyl alcohol 134-5
biotin 79, 80
blood pressure tablets 109
British Journal of Dermatology 34
British Medical Journal 151, 152
British Society for Allergy and
  Environmental Medicine 35,
  38, 61, 177-8
British Society for Nutritional
  Medicine 170
Brostoff, Dr Jonathon 34, 163

Campbell, Dr G.W., 9-10
Candida albicans (thrush) 11, 64-84

caprylic acid 70, 78, 80, 84
carbohydrates 70, 77, 91
Carroll, Dr Murray 153
Carroll, Dr R.A. 35
case histories
  ankylosing spondylitis 10-20, 19-20,
    90-1
  inhaled allergies 59-63
  intestinal candidiasis 81-4
  intradermal testing 160-1
  non-specific arthritis 17-19
  osteoarthritis 15-17
  psoriatic arthritis 87-90
  rheumatoid arthritis 19-20
cheeses 125
chemical sensitivity 20
  and arthritis 43-51
  complicated by Candida 83-51
  diagnosis of 48-9
  and elimination diet 105-6
chemicals
  and additives 46-8
  in food 45-8, 168, 171-2
  inhaled 45
chlorine 16-17, 47
climate, effect of 58-9, 93, 106, 107,
  185
Clinical Allergy 150, 163
Clinical Ecology 34, 35, 40, 164
clinical trials
  of allergy 149-58
  design of 157
  in environmental units 153-6
  in inhaled allergy 162-4
  of neutralization 159-67
  in sublingual provocation 164-7
Coca, Dr Arthur F. 23-4
colitis 159
Committee on Safety in Medicines
  133, 134
Conte, Dr A. 165
contraceptive pill 66, 68, 109
corn 12, 26, 52, 170, 171
  foods containing 127-8
cortisone 11, 13, 17, 49, 60, 62, 66,
  68, 108, 173, 174
cost 11, 12, 37, 102, 142-3, 184
crystal arthritis (gout) 98-9
cyclic food allergies 28-9
cytotoxic testing 37-8

Darlington, Dr Gail 34, 156

desensitization 12, 40
  food 29, 32, 131-43
  incremental 132
  safety of treatment 132-3
diagnosis
  chemical sensitivity 48-9
  of intestinal candidiasis 67-9
  and skin-testing 140-2
Dieppe, Dr Paul 13
diet
  anti-Candida 71-4, 86, 87, 88
  elimination 102-30
  lack of varied 168, 170-1
  low-risk allergy, 15-16, 17, 47, 49,
    54, 56, 109-10
  rotary diversified 29-32
  varied 29, 32, 125
disease-modifying drugs 13, 49, 108
doctors, attitude of 10, 11, 27, 177-8
drug therapy 13
drugs 136-7
  anti-inflammatory 62
  antibiotics 66, 68, 69, 77-8
  aspirin 13, 109
  cortisone-derived 11
  disease-modifying 13, 49, 108
  and elimination diet 107-8
  foodstuffs contained in 107-8
  for intestinal candidiasis 74-8, 80
  non-steroid anti-inflammatory 13,
    108, 151, 154
  side-effects of 13

Eaton, Dr Keith 47
Ebringer, Dr Alan 91-2
echo effect 113
eczema 34, 65, 105, 164
eggs 12, 24-5, 170, 171
elimination diet 11, 17-18, 28, 35-6,
  40, 60, 63, 83, 102-30, 150,
  186
  and chemical sensitivity 105-6
  and drugs 107-9
  effects of 111-12
  emotional reactions to 111
  foods not included 123-5
  and inhaled allergies 106-7
  preparation for 103-9
  Stage I 109-14
  Stage II 114-18
  Stage III 118-20
  Stage IV 120-3

endorphins 42
environmental control units 10-11, 12, 22, 49-51, 65
  trials in 153-6
environmental factors 9, 18
enzyme potentiated desensitization 40-1, 143
ethylene gas 46, 48
evaluation of elimination diet
  stage I 112-14
  stage II 117-18
  stage III 120
  stage IV 122-3
exclusion diets, history of 21-2

fasting 10, 11, 51, 154-5
fatigue 26, 43, 45, 93, 103, 115
Feingold diet 47
Finn, Dr Ronald 33, 164, 184
fixed food allergies 28
food allergy
  and alcoholism 53-4
  and arthritis 21-43
  in children 34
  complicated by Candida 83-4
  cyclic 28-29
  fixed 28
  history of 21-4
  masking 24-7
  tests for 35-40
  treatment for 40-2
food colourants 47-8
food families 29-32, 56
food mixtures 29, 171
foods implicated 12
foods not in elimiantion diet 123-5
formaldehyde 44, 49, 106, 145, 147-8
Freed, Dr David 167

garlic 79-80
gas 18, 44, 45, 48, 105-6, 117, 145, 146-7
general adaptation syndrome 27-8, 173-4
genetics 97, 99, 100, 169
  and psoriasis 86, 89
glycerine 134
Gold 13, 47, 49, 108, 151, 154
gout 98-9
Graham, Dr Pamela 34
Grant, Dr Ellen 34, 68

headaches 26, 43, 45, 62, 105, 112, 115
heartbeat, rapid 104
Heberden nodes 96
Herxheimer response (die-off reaction) 75-7, 78, 80
Hicklin, Dr. A.J. 35, 150
histamine granules 137, 139
house dust 9, 10, 19, 37, 58, 59, 60, 61, 63, 106-7, 117, 144, 145, 185
house dust mite, 9, 10, 19, 37, 58, 59, 60, 61, 63, 106-7, 117, 144, 145, 163-4, 185
Hughes, Dr Graham 151
Hunter, Dr John 34
hydrocarbons 45, 46, 48-9
hyperactivity, 47, 162

immune system, 11, 41, 49, 66-7,
92, 136-9, 175-6
immunology 23-4, 136-7
Independent, the 91
ingested allergens, reaction to 9, 10
inhaled allergens 19, 36-7
  and arthritis 58-63
  and elimination diet 106-7
  and neutralization injections 132
  reaction to 9, 10
  trials in 162-4
inhaled chemicals 45
intestinal candidiasis 49, 64-84, 146, 168, 172, 185-6
  diagnosis of 67-9
  predisposing factors to 68-9
  symptoms of 69-70
  treatment of 70-81
  see also Candida albicans
intolerance, history of 104
intradermal injections 138
intradermal provocative skin-testing 36, 48, 103
intradermal provocative technique 11, 12, 40, 60
intradermal testing, and neutralization 159-62
irritable bowel syndrome 34, 65, 105

joint pain 15, 16, 17, 19, 26, 61, 88, 89, 108, 112, 113, 151
Journal of Clinical Ecology 153

Ketoconazole (Nizoral) 70, 77, 78, 79, 80, 86, 87, 88
King, Dr D. 165
Kirwan, Dr. J.R. 156
Klebsiella 91-2

Lactobacillus acidophilus 70, 78-9, 80
Lancet, 11-12, 33, 34, 156, 172, 185
language of illness 178-80
Lee, Dr Carlton H. 131-2, 134
Lehman, Dr C. 166
leucotrienes 137
low-risk allergy diet 15-16, 17, 47, 49, 54, 56, 109-10

Maberly, Dr Jonathon, 49, 111
McEwen, Dr Len 35, 40-1, 143, 150
Mackarness, Dr Richard 32-3, 39-40, 48, 54, 100, 170
malt 16, 17
Mandell, Dr Marshal 54, 135-6, 165
Mansfield, Dr J.R. 156
masking 24-7, 28, 52-3, 56, 111-12, 174
mast cells 137, 138
microflora *see* intestinal candidiasis
migraine 34, 62, 65, 105, 112, 159, 161
milk 12, 26, 170, 171
  foods containing 128-9
Miller, Dr Joseph 134, 159, 161, 186
Monro, Dr Jean 34, 49
morning stiffness 26-7, 61
moulds 9, 10, 37, 58, 59, 68, 82, 106-7, 117, 145-6, 185
multiple food sensitivities 122-3, 131

myalgic encephalomyelitis (ME) 175

National Health Service 36, 38, 61, 133
Nature 27
neutralization 36, 131-43
  clinical trials of 159-67
  establishing levels 144-5
  injections 17, 19-20, 60-1, 63
    for inhaled allergens 132
  and intradermal testing 159-62
  therapy 9, 17, 19, 20, 59, 80-1, 88, 118
    administration of 139-40
    disadvantages of 142-3
    how it works 136-9
    to chemicals 144-8
    to inhalants 144-8
neutralizing dose, 48, 131-2, 135, 162
Nizoral 70, 77, 78, 79, 80, 86, 87, 88
non-specific arthritis 9, 49
non-steroid anti-inflammatory drugs 13, 108, 151, 154
nutritional deficiencies 168, 169-70
Nystatin 70, 74-5, 76, 77, 78, 79, 80, 82, 84, 86, 88

obesity 104
oil 44, 45, 145
oleic acid 79, 80
organic food 46, 49, 51, 155
osteoarthritis 9, 82, 95-6

pain, joint 15, 16, 17, 19, 26, 61, 88, 89, 108, 112, 113, 151
paraffin wax 47
Parke, Dr A.L. 151
Penicillamine 13, 49, 108, 151
pesticides 44, 45-6, 47
petrochemicals 48
phenol 49, 106, 147-8
philosophy of New Medicine 182-4
plastics 43, 45
pollens 37, 58
polymyalgia rheumatica 100
potassium bicarbonate 116-17
potatoes 52
Pottenger cat studies 168-9
Prednisolone 151, 154
prick testing 36-7, 144-5
prostaglandins 137
provocation neutralization testing 132
provocative neutralization treatment 40, 132
  safety of 133-4
  technique 134-6
psoriasis 65, 82-3, 85-90
psoriatic arthritis 9, 85-90, 97-8

questionnaire, food allergy 103-5

Radcliffe, Dr Michael 61
radionics 38
Randolph, Dr Theron 22, 27, 28, 32, 34, 35, 43-4, 45, 48, 50, 52, 54, 55, 147, 153, 185
RAST test (Radioallergosorbent Test) 37
Rea, Dr William 35, 50, 153, 161, 172

reintroduction of foods 10, 16, 17, 21, 22, 24, 36, 49, 54, 63, 88, 114-18, 150, 155
  order of 115, 118-20, 120-2
Reiter's disease 97
resistance 65-6, 172-6
rheumatic fever 101
rheumatoid arthritis 9, 13, 21, 34, 49, 60, 62, 83, 93-5
  juvenile 95
  symptoms of 93-4
  tests for 94
rhinitis 19, 24-5, 58, 62, 159, 163
Rinkel, Dr Herbert 24-7
Rinkel hyperacute response 26, 28, 174, 183
Rosenberg, Professor Williams 86-7
rotary diversified diet 29-32
  sample 31
Rowe, Dr Albert 21-2, 24, 150

safety
  of desensitization treatment 132-3
  of Nizoral 77
  of Nystatin 74-5
  of provocative neutralization therapy 133-4
salicylates 151
Scadding, Dr Glenis 163
sedimentation rate 94, 151, 154
Selye, Hans 27-8, 173
septic (bacterial) arthritis 101
side-effects, drugs 13
skin, composition of 137-8
skin-testing 11, 18, 19, 20
  and diagnosis 140-2
  prick tests 36-7, 144-5
sleeping tablets 109
smoking 45, 56-7, 110, 183-4

sodium bicarbonate 110, 116-17
Soothill, Professor 34
soya beans 12, 170, 171
  foods containing 130
stiffness 15, 26-7, 61, 112, 113
subcutaneous injections 132, 139, 140
sublingual drops 132, 139-40, 146
sublingual provocation trials 164-7
sublingual testing 39-40
sugar 12, 52, 56-7, 66, 69, 70, 73, 82, 170, 171
sulphur dioxide 46-7
Sunday Times, 13
sweating bouts 104
swelling 15, 17, 61, 88, 89, 104, 108, 112, 113, 151
symptoms 15, 17, 18, 103-5, 151, 159
  and chemical sensitivity 43, 45
  deterioration of 26
  improvement in 10, 18, 84
  of intestinal candidiasis 69-70
  psychological 165
  reduction in 102-3
synthetic ethanol 48, 106
systemic lupus erythematosus 99-100

T-lymphocytes 67, 84, 175
tests
  for allergy 35-40
  foods 116-17
  re-testing 116-17, 142, 163-4
  for rheumatoid arthritis 94
therapy *see* drug therapy; neutralization therapy
thrush *see* Candida albicans; intestinal candidiasis

tolerance, development of 28-9, 171
treatment
  Candida albicans 67
  for food allergies 40-2
  of intestinal candidiasis 70-81
  trials *see* clinical trials
Trowbridge, Dr J.P. 67
Truss, Dr Orion 64-5, 85-6, 146, 185
types of arthritis 93-101
  see also under individual names

ulcerative colitis 40-1
urticaria 65, 105, 164

viral arthritis 100-1
von Pirqet, Clement 22-3

Walker, Morton 67
water
  spring 16, 110
  tap 16, 110
weather, effect of 58-9, 68
wheals 19, 135, 140, 164
wheat 12, 16, 17, 26, 52, 171
  foods containing 127
Williams, Dr R. 152
withdrawal response 28
  classic 16, 26, 63, 108, 112-13
  severe 17-18, 88, 89

X-rays 95, 96, 97

yeast 12, 26, 52, 53-4, 55, 66, 69, 73, 74, 170
  foods containing 129-30

Zeller, Dr Michael 21, 22, 27, 150

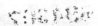